Plain   Words

About

AIDS

Second   Edition

With A Glossary Of Related Terms

Edited by
Wm. Hovey Smith

P L A I N   W O R D S   A B O U T   A I D S
Second Edition

Edited By

Wm. Hovey Smith

Based On

Presentments of the 1986
International Conference on AIDS
June 23-25, Paris, France
Presentments of the 1986
Seventh National Lesbian-Gay Health Conference
March 13-15 Washington, D.C.
Presentments of the 1985
International Conference on AIDS
April 14-17, Atlanta, Georgia
Releases from the
Centers For Disease Control
June 5, 1981 - July 4, 1986
Articles from the
National Wire Services
Through October 20, 1986

WHITEHALL PRESS-BUDGET PUBLICATIONS
Whitehall
Rte. 1   Box 603
Sandersville, Georgia 31082

ISBN 0-916565-09-2

PLAIN WORDS ABOUT AIDS

TABLE OF CONTENTS

TABLES

page

ILLUSTRATIONS

page

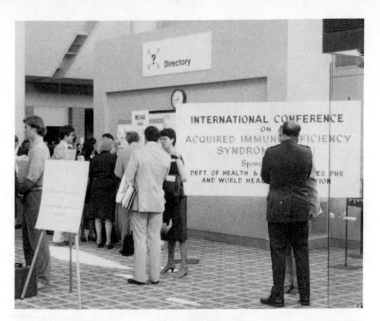

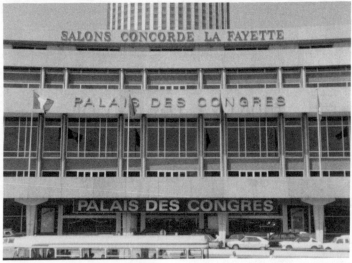

Figure 1. The first International Conference on AIDS held in Atlanta, Georgia in April, 1985, and the second held in Paris, France in June, 1986, provided forums for AIDS-researchers from around the world to pool their knowledge and efforts to defeat this deadly syndrome. (Top) World Congress Center, Atlanta. (Bottom) Palais des Congress, Paris.

EDITOR'S PREFACE

TWO MILLION AMERICANS and five-to-10 million people throughout the world are now suspected to be infected with the AIDS virus, and AIDS is no longer restricted to minority groups (1, 5). These conditions arose because the virus may cause no symptoms for eight years or longer; and those who contracted AIDS during a sexual contact, blood transfusion, or self-administered drug injection years ago are presumed to be capable of infecting others while showing no evidence of ill health (1).

Heralded as the "gay plague" by some less than responsible members of the press and announced from fundamentalist pulpits as "God's vengeance" on those whose sexual practices deviated from the norm, AIDS is neither a plague visited on homosexuals nor a manifestation of God's will. It is an infectious viral disease having serious consequences, like polio; and, as in the case of polio, a cure will be found for AIDS. In the meantime, there is a need to take prudent precautions and logical actions -- not indulgences into hysteria.

AIDS has been designated the Number 1 public health priority by the United States Department of Health and Human Services. Hundreds of thousands of research hours and over $400 million have been spent by the department since 1981 to attempt to solve the medical and social problems presented by this syndrome (3, 6), and large research commitments have also been made by France, Germany, England, Italy, and Sweden.

The April, 1985, International Conference on AIDS in Atlanta sponsored by the United States Department of Health and the World Health Organization provided the first opportunity for over 2,400 scientist working on different aspects of the AIDS problem to exchange information (4). This book is largely based on the 418 papers and posters presented at this conference with modifications and additions to incorporate new information derived from more than 900 presentations from the Second International Conference on AIDS held in June,

1

1986, in Paris <u>and</u> an additional 100 presentments given during the Seventh Annual Lesbian and Gay Health Conference held in Washington, D.C., in March, 1986. Information was also incorporated from several papers delivered during the Second World Congress of Sexually Transmitted Diseases which immediately followed the Paris AIDS conference.

Because most of these papers have several authors and some will be published in volumes of proceedings, the person who delivered the paper is referenced as the author along with the paper or poster's title to enable the reader to identify the source document. The professional titles of those delivering the presentations have been omitted because many were not included in the source materials from the conferences.

This author takes no credit for the research findings of others, but only for compiling these findings into a coherent work that is more understandable to most readers than the original technical documents. In any such work, there is the opportunity for errors of commission and omission, and for these the author takes full responsibility. Comments on this book are welcome and may be sent to the publisher.

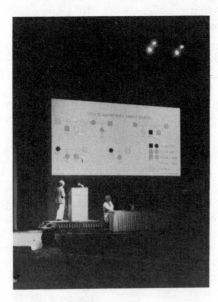

Figure 2. Presentation by Sivita Pahwa of the North Shore Univ. Hospital of Manhasset, N. Y., titled, "Spectrum of HTLV-III Infection in Children." First International Conference on AIDS, Atlanta, Ga., 1985.

It is recognized that there are many scientific and

sociologic discoveries to be made about AIDS. Some perplexing problems will remain unresolved for years, despite rapid progress being made in other aspects of AIDS research. Nonetheless, because of the rate at which new discoveries are being made, it can be anticipated that this book will soon be obsolete; and revised editions will incorporate new information as it becomes available.

This book should be considered a work in progress that will come to its logical conclusion when a cure for AIDS is developed. No one will now speculate when a cure might be discovered or a vaccine produced to protect the uninfected portion of the population.

Some previously unmet needs were recognized when this book was written. One of these was for a simplified glossary of medical terms related to AIDS and associated diseases. From what began as a two-to-three page addendum grew to a 40-page supplement. Although an attempt has been made to reduce the technical language to a minimum, the reader is encouraged to utilize the glossary to help interpret this or other works on AIDS.

Because AIDS is predominately transmitted by sexual activity, it is necessary to define some sexual practices that some readers will find offensive. These practices are not advocated or glamorized, but it is necessary that no doubt remain in the reader's mind as to what is being discussed.

This book was not written to be a self-diagnosis manual and its use for that purpose is discouraged. If a person has reason to believe that he has AIDS or is at risk, he should consult his physician. There are diseases that produce symptoms which mimic AIDS. In addition, the numerous opportunistic infections to which AIDS-infected individuals are predisposed have their own symptomatologies. In one study, gay men with no overt symptoms of AIDS were asked to predict if their test results for the AIDS virus would be positive or negative. When these responses were compared with the test results, the individual's predictions were found to be unreliable (4).

Thanks are due to the numerous researchers, both

named and unnamed, who did the painstaking work on which this book is based, to members of the Centers for Disease Control and National Institutes of Health who extended their willing cooperation, to the World Federation of Hemophilia in the Federal Republic of Germany for furnishing bibliographical information, and to The National Lesbian and Gay Health Foundation, Inc. of Washington D.C. for providing information on gay lifestyles.

A special acknowledgement is given to the numerous volunteers who have participated in AIDS research projects, even at the risk of divulging the most intimate details of their lives.

Only by coincidence might the contents of this book reflect the official positions of any of the above-named organizations, and no endorsement of this work by these organizations is implied.

PREFACE TO THE SECOND EDITION

THE SECOND INTERNATIONAL CONFERENCE ON AIDS held at Paris in 1986 marked five years since the first cases of AIDS-related opportunistic infections were identified in California. This conference documented the steady advance of scientific and sociologic progress, but failed to present any spectacular breakthroughs in combating the syndrome.

At least five different approaches are now being tested which may lead for a vaccine, but the general opinions of leading researchers in the field, like Robert C. Gallo of the National Institutes of Health, is that large scale use of a vaccine is years, and perhaps a decade or more, away.

Gallo remarked during a news conference, "I refuse to speculate when a vaccine will be developed. We are now taking the first steps of outlining approaches, in vitro trials, and animal testing. Only when trials of an agent in an appropriate animal host have begun can one reasonably speculate when these trials will be completed

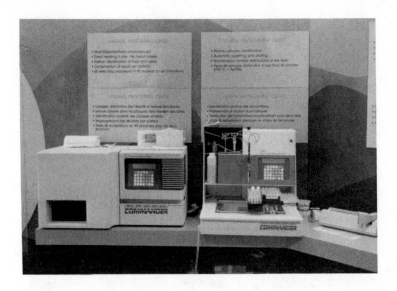

Figure 3.   Techniques for rapid sample processing, such
       as these Abbott instruments exhibited at the Second
       International Conference on AIDS in Paris, have
       enabled large-scale screening of donated blood in
       industrialized countries. The international confer-
       ences on AIDS have become increasingly important
       trade shows for new equipment.

(and if they are successful) what the approximate time
might be for production of a vaccine (7)."
       Only one human vaccine, rabies, is known that will
protect an individual who is already infected with a
disease (8).   Even with the development of a vaccine to
protect the uninfected portion of the population, the
vast reservoir of cases who are already carrying the
virus will continue to present new cases of AIDS for
years after the vaccine has been generally administered.
       A large number of agents with known or suspected
antiviral activity are being tested for their effectiveness against AIDS, and now that the structure and methods
of activity of the virus are somewhat known, drugs are
being sought or designed to interrupt the virus at criti-

cal stages in its life cycle.

An analogy can be drawn between the risks of treating syphilis with mercury and arsenic compounds at some risks to the patient with antiviral drugs which often provoke toxic reactions. Using new drugs in humans, after they have demonstrated their effectiveness in animal trials, must be done with extreme care to detect the earliest signs of adverse effects. Such testing must proceed slowly until enough information has been assembled from a sufficiently large population to determine the appropriate, safe dosage of the drug.

One might sum up the findings of the Second International Conference on AIDS as follows:

1. AIDS is rapidly becoming a world-wide epidemic and no sex, nationality or ethnic group is immune from infection.

2. AIDS is spread through heterosexual contact, but at a slower rate than through homosexual contact with exchange of body fluids and IV drug use.

3. The number of cases of AIDS will continue to increase even though a slowing of the rate of increase will probably be seen in the United States during the next few years because of the withdrawal of contaminated blood products and a decrease in new infections among homosexuals due to the general adoption of safer sex practices.

4. AIDS is principally spread through sexual activity, use of contaminated needles, and blood products.

5. Numerous case studies have demonstrated that AIDS is NOT readily spread among family members in a home setting even when one family member has the disease and many common household items are shared.

6. The risk of catching AIDS through casual contact with an infected individual is so small as to be almost nonexistent.

7. AIDS is uncommonly, and perhaps not, transmitted through saliva, tears, or sweat in the absence of accompaning blood; and not commonly through mother's milk.

8. There is no proof that AIDS is transmitted by vectors such as mosquitos, and much anecdotal evidence to suggest that it is not.

9. No cofactors have been proved that appear to predetermine who will progress from seropositivity to full-blown AIDS, although suggestions were frequently made that reinoculation with different variant of the AIDS virus or other venereal diseases may be important.

10. Social support of AIDS patients, their families, and lovers is as important as the clinical treatment of the disease.

11. The legal and civil rights aspects of AIDS are still in flux with continuing conflicts between the needs to protect society and to preserve civil liberties, particularly in legislatures of nations and states where the first AIDS cases are now developing.

12. Education remains the most effective tool in slowing the rate of spread of AIDS; but because of the years-long incubation period significant drops in the rate of increase of AIDS cases cannot be expected until years after the emplacement of an effective program.

13. The time to began an education program is as the first cases of AIDS occur in a nation or state, not when the problem reaches crisis proportions, and such a program must reach all sexually active members of the population and not just targeted "risk groups."

14. Educational programs must take into account the different social, economic, and religious values held in the population which these programs serve.

15. Because AIDS is not a single disease, but a syndrome of diseases, much diversity is seen throughout the world in the prevalence of different opportunistic infections.

16. The treatment and consequences of AIDS will demand much from the world's health and social care systems for decades, and organizers of AIDS programs should realize that the programs they design may be in use beyond the year 2050.

17. Task forces and networking programs to bring together groups of diverse interest, offer the best ap-

proach to the AIDS dilemma provided information can be easily exchanged to prevent needless duplications of efforts.

Wm. Hovey Smith

---

1. Curran, James W., 198A, The epidemiology and prevention of AIDS: Centers for Disease Control, Atlanta, Georgia, International Conference on AIDS, Atlanta, Georgia.

2. Holland, Jimmie C.B., 1985, Psycosocial and neuropsychiatric sequeiae of AIDS and AIDS related disorders: Memorial Sloan-Kettering Cancer Center, New York, New York, International Conference on AIDS, Atlanta, Georgia.

3. Noble, Gary R., 1985, Program chairman, opening session: International Conference on AIDS, Atlanta, Georgia.

4. McCutchan, J. Allen, 1985, Implications of HTLV-III antibody testing for gay men: Univ. Calif., San Diego, International Conference on AIDS, Atlanta, Georgia.

5. Mahler, H., 1986, World Health Organization's program on AIDS: Opening session, Second International Conference on AIDS, Paris, France.

6. MacDonald, Gary, 1986, The politics of AIDS: Seventh National Lesbian and Gay Health Conference, Washington, D.C.

7. Gallo, Robert C., 1986, Press conference, June 25: Second International Conference on AIDS, Paris, France.

8. Zinkernagel, Rolf, M., 1986, Why could AIDS agents be successful in evading immune surveillance?: Zurich Institute for Pathology, Second International Conference on AIDS, Paris, France.

American College of Physicians, 1985, Annals of internal medicine; including the international conference on acquired immunodeficiency syndrome: November, vol. 103, no. 5, pp. 653-781.

THE BODY'S DEFENSE SYSTEMS

A DEFENSE IN DEPTH is how a military-minded person might describe the human body's mechanisms for combating diseases, a system so carefully designed with so many interrelated components that it would appear almost impossible for an invading organism to penetrate the body's physical, chemical, and biochemical barriers. Any general would be proud of designing such a system to protect his homeland.

Every day the body is exposed to thousands of microorganisms, some of which have the potential for causing serious diseases. Other protozoans, fungi, and viruses happily utilize the human body to provide food, shelter, and protection as they complete their life cycles. While it may seem strange to realize that the body might be home to more than a dozen different creatures living within it, such is the case. They have become so used to their environment that they often form a community which feeds on body waste products and leave the body alone. In fact, some of them may be helpful by attacking competing organisms before they have a chance to do harm.

Each person collects his own microorganisms, or "bugs," as he goes through life. Some are fairly wide spread, like the fungus that causes thrush; but others are geographically restricted like Histoplasma capsulatum, the fungus which causes the disease histoplasmosis. Histoplasma is native to parts of the Ohio and Mississippi valleys, parts of New England and the Caribbean. It is not normally found elsewhere, unless infected soils are transported.

A newborn begins his "bug" collecting immediately after birth. When exposed to a new microbe, he may come down with a mild fever, diarrhea, or other symptoms, depending on the infecting agent; but for the most part, these are dismissed as the usual childhood diseases unless the symptoms become severe. After the initial infection is over and the "bug" has made himself a home in the body, it and its descendents may reside there quite happily for years. Only when an unusual condition occurs such as when competing organisms are killed off by an antibiotic, its food supply becomes suddenly more abundant, or the body's natural immunization system fails, do most of the body's cohabitants cause any problems.

The first problem facing an invading organism is how to get into the body. The skin, with its constantly regenerating layers of tissue, does its job of defeating invading agents very well. It is flexible, resilient, and reasonably tear-resistant. If the skin remains intact, an invading agent can only enter through the nose, mouth, ears, eyes, anus, and penis or vagina -- all of which have separate protective mechanisms to capture, kill, eject, or digest foreign agents.

Say, for example, that a healthy person is exposed to a flu virus. Because of its very small size, too small to be observed with an ordinary optical microscope and much smaller than human cells, the body has difficulty in trapping and expelling the virus as it can more easily enter cells which larger organisms cannot. If ingested through the nose, the virus is exposed to a convoluted surface lined with sticky mucus in the sinuses. Normally, mucus is an efficient filter and traps, like flypaper, most solid material.

The problem that the flu virus has is to penetrate the walls of a cell, as viruses must pirate the reproductive ability of a living cell to reproduce. Once a suitable cell has been penetrated, viral reproduction starts, new viruses are made, and they work their way into the throat.

Assuming that these conditions did occur, symptoms like nasal congestion, a runny nose, mild fever, and a sore throat might be soon noted, confirming that the body is falling back on its second and third lines of defenses.

Chemical signals activating the body's lymphatic system are sent as soon as the invading virus enters the host cell. Previously, the body's defense system had

been a passive, barrier-erection sort of resistance, but
now the body is preparing to do battle in an active,
aggressive manner by seeking and destroying foreign organisms.

The first aggressive reaction might be from a portion of the body's lymphatic system known as the reticuloendothelial system. This system contains several
types of scavenging, or phagocytic, cells which envelop
and consume foreign organisms. Among these are the macrophage cells, a type of white blood cell or leukocyte.
These are attracted to the site of the infection by T-
cells, which are products of the thymus gland.

There are two types of T-cell lymphocytes, designated as T-4 helper cells and T-8 suppressor cells. Both
of the T cells recognize the foreign shape of the invading virus. After adhering to the invading shape, the T-4
cells send a chemical signal to attract nearby macrophages. In addition, some T-cells contain a toxin, a
poison, which may be used to kill the cell containing the
virus.

Some very fine balances are struck by the activities
of the T-cells. They must destroy the invading organisms
and the infected cells, but leave untouched the nearby
healthy cells. That task requires a high degree of discriminatory ability, like deciding who is and is not the
enemy in a guerilla war; but, for the most part, the T-
cells do a good job. At times, and for reasons yet
unknown, the T-cells will attack some group of the body's
cells that are apparently healthy; and the body will
develop an autoimmune disease. Rheumatoid arthritis is
such a disease where the body's immune system is attacking connective tissues in the bone joints.

Meanwhile, back at the battlefield, plasma cells in
the blood have begun to produce antibodies that specifically attack the irritating substances (antigens) produced by, and on the surface of, the infecting virus.

As the battle continues, there are casualties on
both sides, and dead cells are transported away by the
small vessels of the lymph system or the bloodstream. In
both cases they enter a filter system, either the lymph

nodes or the liver. Some live or only wounded viruses
are likely to be transported to the follicular dendritic
cells of the lymph nodes. In the process of killing these
viruses the lymph glands swell and may become painfully
sore during an infectious episode. Dead cells in the
bloodstream are trapped by the liver which, in turn,
passes the smaller debris onto the kidneys for eventual
discharge from the body in the urine.

Ultimately, the spread of the virus is stopped, the
symptoms of illness pass, and the patient recovers to
have a life-long resistance to reinfection. Immunity to
many infectious diseases is acquired in this manner.

Thus, a single infectious episode localized in the
nostrils and throat elicits a response from the physical
barriers like the mucus linings, chemical responses with
the antitoxins produced to combat it, biochemical responses as by the killer T-cells, transportation through both
the lymphatic and blood systems, filtering, and expulsion
from the body.

By any standards this is a very complex defense
mechanism, but this brief description does not mention
defenses within the cell where a similar round of trapping, encapsulating, and expulsion takes place; special-
ized defenses like tears and ear wax to wash away or trap
foreign particles; the secretions of fluids by the lungs
and coughing to expel these fluids; and other sophisti-
cated plans the body has for neutralizing and ridding
itself of invading substances.

The T-4 lymphocytes are key scouts in the body's
array of defenses. Should the thymus no longer be able
to produce this and other lymphocytes, or if the function
of these lymphocytes is impaired, infectious agents have
a head start establishing a foothold.

In AIDS, the T-8, or suppressor, cells, become more
numerous than the T-4 cells because large numbers of T-4
cells are killed by the AIDS virus. The result is that
the suppressor cells outnumber the helper cells by a
margin of more than 2:1. This increased number of T-8
suppressor cells prevents the T-4 cells from combating
infections by sending a false chemical message that the

invading antigen has already been defeated. The imbalance of the T-4 : T-8 ratio can be detected by standard blood analyses and is considered an indicator of the progression of AIDS.

With the protective lymphatic system impaired, the infecting agent can use the vessels that carry the lymphatic fluid as attack routes to infest the body. In the same manner, the bloodstream becomes a carrier of infections which now may become localized in the liver and other organs. Such a cycle of infection may spread very rapidly and, depending on the invading agent, could have deadly results.

Not only does the body fail to respond effectively to new infectious agents, the body's "bugs" find this an opportune time to turn traitor and attack as well. Reoccurrences of diseases like herpes simplex may appear, but with much more serious consequences than ever before. Fungi like Candida albicans may become more active and cause outbreaks of thrush resulting in sore patches and swelling in the mouth and throat. Protozoan like Isospora belli, which have coexisted quite happily in the intestine for years, may now cause a severe diarrhea known as isosporiasis.

Those whose immune system is severely deficient may have simultaneous or sequential attacks of several AIDS-related diseases, which not only leads to the discomfort of the patient but also increases the difficulty of treatment. If the body's ability to produce white blood cells cannot be restored, some white blood cells can be introduced back into the body by transfusion, but unfortunately not the T-cells because they are so finely attuned to a given body that they are rejected when another person's blood is used.

Most bacterial and protozoan infections can be treated with antibiotics, but these drugs have no effect on virus infections. Drugs powerful enough to treat virus infections often have very severe side effects. Some are cytotoxic or cell killers and while they may kill the cell containing the virus or cancer, a lot of healthy cells may also be injured or destroyed. Cytotoxic drugs are usually given only in the case of chemotherapy for life-threatening diseases.

When antiviral agents have been developed for AIDS, they can be introduced into the bloodstream; but unless such agents are specifically designed to respond to antigens particular to the virus and infected T-4 cells, they may also destroy healthy T-cells.

A common misconception about AIDS is that this disability of the body's immune system makes a person likely to succumb to every infectious agent to which he may be exposed. This is not the case except perhaps during the final stages of AIDS. Although the immune system is impaired, some immunities remain functional through most of the progression of AIDS. There are a particular set of diseases associated with AIDS. While these appear numerous, they are a relatively small number when compared to the much larger number of infectious diseases in humans.

Many visits made to doctors' offices by AIDS patients and the "worried well" are not related to illness, but are caused by the psychological needs of the patients for support. Self-education and seeking social support from volunteer and public agencies can prevent many unnecessary visits to doctors and permit physicians to spend more time treating those with serious medical needs.

AIDS, WHAT IT IS AND IS NOT

DETERMINING THE CAUSE of any infectious disease is one of the first steps that must be taken in order to combat it.   It's like attempting to find out which dish served in a restaurant was the cause of food poisoning. If everyone who ate the salmon balls subsequently devel- oped food poisoning, that would be convincing circum- stantial evidence that the salmon balls were responsible.

To carry this analogy further, consider that some of the guests who ate the salmon balls had no symptoms of food poisoning; that others, some of whom ate the suspect salmon balls and some did not, developed infections of the lungs and eyes or cancers of the skin, while still others had symptoms to appear months after they dined at the restaurant.   Were all of these symptoms related to the same agent?   Were the salmon balls the exclusive method of transmission?   Why was the onset of symptoms delayed in some cases and not in others?

These would be the questions that any person in- vestigating this hypothetical incidence of food poisoning would ask, and these were some of the questions that immediately presented themselves in 1981 when the first cases of the syndrome of diseases that was later named AIDS were reported.

Since, at first, the cause of the syndrome was not known, it had to be described by the characteristic dis- eases which appeared to categorize it.   It was like saying, "We don't know what causes AIDS, but if a patient has one of the following diseases which indicates a cellular immune deficiency and has an apparent immune deficiency with no other identifiable cause, we'll say that he has AIDS." So, it developed in 1981 and 1982 that a group of diseases were necessary to define the syn- drome; and even when the causative virus was identified in 1984, it was still the expression of characteristic disease/s that was used to diagnose AIDS. When the def-

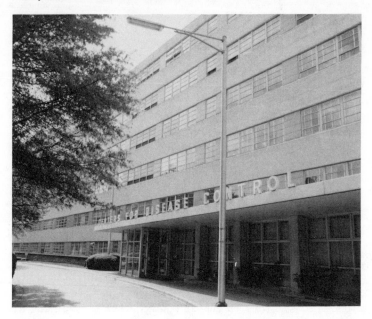

Figure 4. The Centers for Disease Control in Atlanta, Georgia. This agency, which is a part of the Public Health Service of the United States Department of Health and Human Services, monitors outbreaks of unusual and contagious diseases worldwide and is an important agency for gathering information on the spread of AIDS. CDC photo.

inition was revised in a CDC release on June 28, 1985, the syndrome was still defined "to include only the more severe manifestations of HTLV-III/LAV infection" -- not just the presence of antibodies to the AIDS virus in the blood or identification of the virus in tissue cultures. The official CDC definition is given below:

CENTERS FOR DISEASE CONTROL CASE DEFINITION OF AIDS

For the limited purposes of epidemiologic sur- veillance, CDC defines a case of "the acquired im- mune deficiency syndrome" (AIDS) as a person who has had:

I. a reliably diagnosed disease that is at least moderately indicative of an underlying cellular immune deficiency, but who, at the same time, has had:

II. no known underlying cause of cellular immune deficiency nor any other cause of reduced resistance reported to be associated with that disease.

This general definition is made more specific by the CDC by a listing of the diseases and manifestations of these diseases required for a diagnosis of AIDS. All of these diseases were known prior to the AIDS epidemic. They all may have other causes than AIDS. Only if one of these diseases is present and only if there is no other cause of the immune deficiency can the case be diagnosed as AIDS. Nowhere in either the past or present CDC definitions of AIDS is the presence of the AIDS virus or antibodies the exclusive means of diagnosis.

The CDC definition of AIDS continues:

1. Disease at least moderately indicative of underlying cellular immune deficiency:
These are listed below in five etiological (causative agent) categories: A. protozoal and helminthic, B. fungal, C. bacterial, D. viral and E. cancer. Within each category, the diseases are listed in alphabetical order. "Disseminated infection" refers to involvement of liver, bone marrow, or multiple organs, not simply involvement of lungs and multiple lymph nodes. The required diagnostic methods with positive results are shown in parentheses.

A. Protozoal and Helminthic Infections:
1. Cryptosporidiosis, intestinal, causing diarrhea for over one month, (on histology or stool microscopy);
2. Pneumocystis carinii pneumonia, (on

histology, or microscopy of a "touch" preparation or bronchial washing);

3. Strongyloidosis, causing pneumonia,
central nervous system infection, or disseminated infection, (on histology);

4. Toxoplasmosis, causing pneumonia or
central nervous system infection (on histology
or microscopy of a "touch" preparation);

B. Fungal Infections:
1. Candidiasis, causing esophagitis (on
histology, or microscopy of a "wet" preparation
from the esophagus, or endoscopic findings of
white plaques on an erythematous mucosal base);

2. Cryptococcosis, causing central nervous system, or disseminated infection (on
culture, antigen detection, histology, or India
ink preparation of CSF);

C. Bacterial Infections:
1. "Atypical" mycobacteriosis (species
other than tuberculosis or lepra), causing
disseminated infection (on culture);

D. Viral Infections:
1. Cytomegalovirus, causing pulmonary,
gastrointestinal tract, or central nervous system infection (on histology);

2. Herpes simplex virus, causing chronic
mucocutaneous infection with ulcers persisting
more than one month, or pulmonary, gastrointestinal tract, or disseminated infection (on
culture, histology, or cytology);

3. Progressive multifocal leukoencephalopathy (presumed to be caused by Papovavirus)
(on histology);

E. Cancer:
1. Kaposi's sarcoma ((KS) (on histology);
2. Lymphoma limited to the brain (on his-

tology).

The CDC definition of AIDS then lists the known causes of reduced resistance which the definition excludes as being related to AIDS. These are; (1) Patients undergoing medical treatment for cancer in which their immune system is purposefully suppressed. If immune suppression-related diseases are contracted within a month of treatment, they are not considered to be related to AIDS unless the patient has a positive test for the AIDS virus. (2) Widely spread cancer of the lymphatic system which reduces the body's resistance to infections. (3) Kaposi's sarcoma in patients over 60 years old at diagnosis (patients in which this type of cancer is most often seen). (4) Newborns who have toxoplasmosis, cytomegalovirus, or herpes simplex contracted before their bodies were capable of building their own immune systems. (5) Genetic causes of defects in the immune system such as thymic dysplasia or an immune deficiency atypical of AIDS such as hypogammaglobulinemia (1).

REVISED DEFINITION OF AIDS

After consideration of the recommendations of the Conference of State and Territorial Epidemiologists (CSTE) at their 1985 meeting in Madison, Wisconsin, the CDC adopted the recommendations of the conference that some changes be made in the case definition of AIDS. These changes were officially reported in the CDC weekly mortality report dated June 28, 1985. Appropriate sections of the report are reproduced below.

The CSTE approved the following resolutions:
1. That the case definition of AIDS used for national reporting continue to include only the more severe manifestations of HTLV-III/LAV infection, and
2. that CDC develop more inclusive definitions and classifications of HTLV-III/LAV infection for diagnosis, treatment, and prevention, as well as for

epidemiologic studies and special surveys, and

3. that the following refinements be adopted in the case definition of AIDS used for reporting.

a. In the absence of the opportunistic diseases required by the current case definition, any of the following diseases will be considered indicative of AIDS if the patient has a positive serologic or virologic test for HTLV-III/LAV;

(1) disseminated histoplasmosis (not confined to lungs or lymph nodes) diagnosed by culture, histology, or antigen detection;

(2) isosporiasis, causing chronic diarrhea (over 1 month), diagnosed by histology or stool microscopy;

(3) bronchial or pulmonary candidiasis, diagnosed by microscopy or by presence of characteristic white plaques grossly on the bronchial mucosa (not by culture alone);

(4) non-Hodgkin's lymphoma of high-grade pathologic type (diffuse, undifferentiated) and of B-cell or unknown immunological phenotype, diagnosed by biopsy;

(5) histologically confirmed Kaposi's sarcoma in patients who are 60 years old or older when diagnosed.

b. In the absence of the opportunistic diseases required by the current case definition, a histologically confirmed diagnosis of chronic lymphoid interstitial pneumonitis in a child (under 13 years of age) will be considered indicative of AIDS unless test(s) for HTLV-III/LAV are negative.

c. Patients who have a lymphoreticular malignancy diagnosed more than 3 months after the diagnosis of an opportunistic disease used as a marker for AIDS will no longer be excluded as AIDS cases.

d. To increase the specificity of the case definition, patients will be excluded as AIDS cases if they have a negative result on testing for serum antibody to HTLV-III/LAV, have no other type of HTLV-III/LAV test with a positive result, and do not have a low number of T-helper lymphocytes or a low ratio of T-helper to T-suppressor lymphocytes. In the absence of test results, patients satisfying all other criteria in the definition will continue to be included.

CLASSIFICATION OF AIDS

Two systems have been developed for the classification of AIDS, one by the CDC and another at the Walter Reed Hospital. In commenting on the use of the classification, the May 23, 1986, issue of the Morbidity and Mortality Weekly Report, the CDC states, "The classification system applies only to patients diagnosed as having HTLV-III/LAV infection. Classification in a particular group is not explicitly intended to have prognostic significance, nor to designate severity of illness. However, classification in the four principal groups, I-IV, is hierarchical in that persons classified in a particular group should not be reclassified in a preceding group if clinical findings resolve, since clinical improvement may not accurately reflect changes in the severity of the underlying disease (25)."

The CDC classification is designed to facilitate the reporting of AIDS cases and allow additional information to be obtained about individual AIDS cases. The Walter Reed classification reaches further back to the point of exposure and then continues to classify progressively worsening symptomatologies (26). Both classifications imply a progressive worsening of the disease. Might not the subscript "r" also be used in these classifications fications to denote remission and the subscript "c" to denote cure and offer a hint of hope? One day remissions and cures will be commonplace. As it will be just as important to track the rate of cures then as the rate of

TABLE 1. Summary of AIDS classification systems

CDC

Group I.	Acute infection
Group II.	Asymptomatic infection
Group III.	Persistent generalized lymphadenopathy
Group 1V.	Other diseases

Subgroup A. Constitutional disease
        B. Neurologic disease
        C. Secondary infectious diseases
    Category C-1. Specified secondary infectious
                    diseases in CDC surveillance
                    definition for AIDS
           C-2 Other specific secondary
                    infectious diseases
        D. Secondary cancers
        E. Other conditions

Walter Reed

WR 0.	High risk exposure
WR 1.	Asymptomatic infection
WR 2.	Chronic lymphadenopathy
WR 3.	Subclinical T helper cell depletion
WR 4.	Clinical defects in delayed hypersensitivity
WR 5.	Oral candidiasis or anergy
WR 6.	Invasive opportunistic infections

---

of infections now, why not admit that possibility into
the classifications and not have to modify them later?

AIDS-RELATED DISEASES

Some of the diseases mentioned in the CDC definition of AIDS are opportunistic infections caused by a virus, bacteria, fungus, protozoan, or worm, while others are cancers. For reasons that are not entirely evident, this particular group of 12 diseases has a strong prevalence in AIDS patients. The two diseases that are most commonly observed in AIDS patients are the cancer, Kaposi's sarcoma, and <u>Pneumocystis</u> <u>carinii</u> pneumonia. Two or more of the diseases mentioned in the CDC definition, as well as other diseases may occur simultaneously, which complicates diagnosis.

In addition to these diseases, the AIDS virus has been linked with a series of progressively severe mental disorders caused by the virus infecting the brain in some cases. These symptoms include forgetfulness, inability to concentrate, paranoia, neuroses, and global distress. According to the researchers, a general progression in the severity of these symptoms was observed in some cases; but other researchers disagreed on whether these symptoms were invariably progressive or if periods of remission occurred (2).

Organically caused mental illnesses associated with venereal diseases are well known; i.e., the progressive mental deterioration of syphilitic patients. Until penicillin was used for treating syphilitics, they were the largest group of patients in many mental hospitals.

An unanswered question is if AIDS-related mental illnesses are reversible and, if so, at what stage? In the case of victims of syphilis, mild brain damage may be reversible; but profound brain damage is not. A likely speculation is that the nation's mental institutions will have an influx of patients with AIDS-caused mental disorders even after a cure is found for AIDS.

It is difficult to attempt to distinguish between organic mental disorders and those which might be expected in patients with personal histories of rejection and suppression who are informed that they have an incurable disease. For whichever cause, the psychological comforting of AIDS patients is as important as the medical treatment of their disease (3).

Frequently Observed Diseases

Pneumocystis carinii Pneumonia

Commonly referred to as PCP, Pneumocystis carinii pneumonia is caused by an infection by a protozoan (a single-celled animal). This protozoan may be transmitted by the fluids coughed up by the patient. Respiratory isolation is recommended to prevent the spread of the vector to other patients with immune-suppressed systems.

PCP is the most frequently diagnosed infection in AIDS patients, with up to 75 percent of AIDS patients reporting the disease during their course of illness, (4), and it is one of the most common causes of death. In a 1984 study of over 100 patients of the New York University Medical Center, 78 percent of the patients overcame their initial infection (5); but the average survival time was reported to be from 7 to 9 months (4).

This disease is treated with a variety of drugs, and reinfections with the pneumonia often reoccur in patients who responded well to initial treatment. The second bout with the disease is more difficult to cure than the first, and many patients who survived the first PCP infection succumbed to the second.

Two partially successful approaches have resulted in an increased survival time for PCP patients. These have been a change of drugs from the first to the second infection and the administration of a maintenance level of a drug to prevent recurrence.

Drugs used for the treatment of PCP include trimethoprim sulfamethoxazole, cotrimoxarole, and pentamidine isethionate. Fansidar, or maintenance treatment with cotrimoxarole, is recommended as a prophylaxis to prevent reinfection. The fansidar prophylaxis was given as one tablet a week with one patient in a limited study having no recurrence of PCP after 20 months (6). Another drug, eflornithine (eflornithine hydrochloride, DFMO), described by J.L.R. Barlow, was found to be effective in controlling the parasite in 26 of 27 patients who did not require respiratory support prior to treatment (27). Toxic reactions to treatment with these drugs are common with changes in the type of drug or the dosage often being required. Some AIDS patients with no previous sensitivity have not been able to tolerate sulfadrugs (7).

The longevity of AIDS patients with PCP has been remarkably increased since the more general adoption of drug therapies and prophylactic treatments designed to stave off reinfections. PCP remains a serious infection associated with AIDS, but infection with PCP is no longer as serious a condition as it was even 12 months ago. Very rapid progress is being made to combat PCP, and for those who can tolerate sulfadrugs, there is the possibility that this disease can be warded off for years.

Mycobacterium avium pneumonia

This bacteria, which is sometimes expressed as Mycobacterium avium-intracellular, is another frequent cause of severe respiratory and disseminated infection in AIDS patients. This disease is often detected on autopsy. In one group of autopsies at the Sloan-Kettering Cancer Center in New York, the bacteria was found in half of the AIDS patients (2). The bacteria may invade most organs of the body, including the respiratory and digestive system. Up to one million colonies per gram of tissue have been recovered from the spleen and liver (8).

Although PCP is the most frequently diagnosed respiratory infection in AIDS patients, Donald A. Armstrong suggested that mycobacterial infections should also be sought because of the virulence and rapid progression of the disease (4). If Mycobacterium avium is detected early, the chance of successful treatment is better (8).

The bacteria is thought to enter the body through the gastrointestinal tract and spread through the lungs, liver, blood, bone marrow, and spleen (9). Drugs given for the disease include ansamycin and cloflazamine with others (quinolones) being investigated (10). Ansamycin has not been shown to be particularly effective in treating this bacterial infection (8). Maintenance therapy is apparently necessary to prevent reinfections (28).

Drugs which have good in-vitro activity against the bacteria include amikacin, clofazimine, dihydromycoplanecin-A, and rifapertine (29). Drugs which C.B. Inderlied of the USC School of Medicine found to be active against some strains in mice were BMY-2814, ciprofloxacin, and imipenem. He recommends a mixed-drug therapy of amikacin, ciprofloxacin, and imipenem or an alternate of amikacin and rifapertine for initial trials in mice (29).

Kaposi's Sarcoma

Kaposi's sarcoma, or KS, occurs in about 30 percent of AIDS patients. This cancer has been found to invade virtually every organ of the body, although it is most commonly, and most obviously, observed on the skin. When present on the exterior of the body, it occurs as a single or series of pink-to-purple masses rising above the skin which may be flat, rounded, or irregular in form. In AIDS-related KS, the trunk, neck, and head appeared to be favored sights for the cancerous masses, although they may occur on the lower limbs (11).

KS occurs in Eastern Europe, Central Africa, and in the Northeast Part of the North American continent. Prior to the AIDS epidemic, it was uncommonly encountered in the United States among elderly men of Eastern European extraction. Although still primarily a disease of men (A few cases in women with AIDS have been reported.), KS in association with AIDS may occur in children as well as men of all ages (11).

The advance of the disease may be rapid or comparatively slow, depending on site of the cancer and the strength of the body's immune system. A patient with KS involving the surface tissues of the body has a better chance of recovery than a patient with KS of the lungs, where survival may be only a few weeks after diagnosis. In following a series of AIDS-related KS cases, Safai reported that 60 percent survived one year and 50 percent had survived two years after treatment.

Cosmetic disfigurements caused by surface eruptions of KS on the face, neck, and particularly on the nose contribute to the psychological distress of AIDS patients. The successful treatment of these obvious cancers can result in considerable benefit to the patient, even though these cancers may not be life-threatening (12).

Drugs used for the treatment of KS include high-dose interferon and vinblastine, which resulted in complete remission of KS in a group of patients at the Anderson Hospital in Houston, Texas (13). In France, W. Rozenbaum reported success in treating KS with Alpha-2 recombinant interferon, but Gamma recombinant interferon was found to be ineffectual in vivo test by S. Miles of the UCLA School of Medicine (30, 31).

Other AIDS-Associated Diseases

Parasitic Infections - Cryptosporidiosis, Strongyloidosis & Toxoplasmosis

Prior to the start of the AIDS epidemic in about 1981 only seven cases of human infection with the parasite Cryptosporidium difficile had been reported. The parasite was known as an infectious agent in reptiles, birds, fish, and mammals. Infection with this protozoan may lead to a life-threatening diarrhea (14). Because the parasite exists world-wide and may infect many animals kept as pets, AIDS patients should avoid keeping reptiles, birds, and fish as pets and avoid contact with the stool of dogs and cats.

A new ELISA test has been developed for cryptosporidiosis which appears to be a reliable test for the presence of this parasite (14). One drug, amproium, has been used by veterinarians to treat animals infected with this parasite (Cuff, 1984). There is, as of June, 1986, no effective human therapy for cryptosporidiosis, but limited success has been obtained with spiramycin or combinations of quinine and clindamycin (32).

Strongyloidosis is an infection with the roundworm, Strongyloides stercoralis, which is native to the Southeastern United States. This worm may cause a massive infection of the lungs leading to pneumonia. The parasite typically enters the body through the skin, reproduces in the intestines, and migrates through the blood vessels to the lungs. As of the time the CDC definition of AIDS was written, no cases of Strongyloidosis had been documented that were associated with AIDS, but this disease was considered likely to be associated with AIDS because of its previous occurrence in cases of immune deficiency. Thiobendazole is the drug typically used to combat this infection.

Toxoplasmosis, the disease produced by the protozoan parasite, <u>Toxoplasma gondii</u>, most frequently attacks the nervous system and may result in brain lesions, encephalitis or myocarditis. These lesions are one apparent cause of the dementia associated with AIDS (15).

Symptoms of dementia include seizure, focal weakness, headache, confusion, psychosis, and lethargy. While not exclusively produced by <u>Toxoplasma gondii</u>, the organism remains a common cause of brain lesions in AIDS patients. A needle biopsy of brain tissue can be used to confirm the presence of the organism where a CAT scan or symptoms of dementia indicate the presence of the lesions or the parasite (16).

Toxoplasmosis is more commonly seen in Central Africa than in North America, but cases have been reported. This disease has been found to respond to treatment with pyrimethamine and sulfadiazine and F. Raffi of the Claude Bernard Hospital reported complete or partial remission in 88.5 percent of 35 patients (33).

<u>Yeast</u> <u>Infections</u> - <u>Candidiasis</u> & <u>Cryptococcosis</u>

Candidiasis, an infection by <u>Candida albicans</u> often called thrush, is frequently seen in AIDS patients. Typically it occurs as white plaque patches in the mouth, but may also spread into the esophagus and the lungs. Treatment for the Candidiasis includes the drugs nystatin, ketoconazole, and amphotericin.

The presence of thrush is often the first signal of an underlying immune deficiency and some centers, such as the Sloan-Kettering Cancer Center in New York, use the presence of thrush as a warning sign of AIDS (17).

Although candidiasis has the potential of disseminating to sites other than the mouth, Armstrong (2) reports that it usually does not spread to other sites unless a passage like a catheter provides an easy entry into the body.

Candidiasis is not restricted to AIDS patients, and this infection has the potential of being transmitted from person to person during dental care. Not only for the prevention of candidiasis, but also for their own protection, the CDC recommends that dentist wear gloves and take other precautions to prevent contracting diseases from, or spreading them to, their patients (34).

The fungicides ketoconozol or amphotericine B (stilbamine and dihydroxystilbamine) have proved effective against candidia of the mouth and esophagus (28).

Cryptococcus neoformans can cause skin ulcers, pneumonia, meningitis, lymphadenopathy, and endocarditis. Once detected the disease must be aggressively treated and treatment must continue indefinitely (2). As it may attack the lungs or the central nervous system, as well as the body's lymphatic system, it is a serious danger to AIDS patients. It is the most common cause of dementia.

Drugs used in therapy for cryptococcosis are amphotericin B and flucytosine, but therapy has been effective in only about 40 percent of cases with frequent relapses being reported (28). Because of the likelihood of relapse, maintenance therapy with amphotericin B or ketoconozol is often used (28).

Fungal Infections - Histoplasmosis, Coccidioidomycosis, Blastomycosis & Aspergillosis

Histoplasma capsulatum, the causative agent of histoplasmosis, is a fungus that occurs naturally in the soils of the Ohio River Valley, Northeast United States and the Caribbean. The presentation of this disease in AIDS patients may occur years after exposure, leading to patients developing histoplasmosis without recent travel to an area where the fungus is native (18). The disease is often mild in individuals with a normal immune system; but in those whose immune system is impaired, it may result in pulmonary infections, ulcers of the gastrointestinal tract, leukopenia, and enlargement of the spleen and liver.

Treatment for histoplasmosis includes the drugs

amphotericin B and ketoconazole. Long term, if not indefinite, treatment is necessary to prevent a relapse.

Coccidioidomycosis also has the potential for spreading to the lungs, lymph nodes, and digestive tract, as well as causing skin lesions and locating in the central nervous system where it can cause meningitis. The fungicides amphotericin and ketoconazole are frequently given in therapy for six months or longer.

Blastomycosis may result in lesions on the skin, in the lungs, and may also disseminate into the muscles, central nervous system, and kidneys. This disease is caused by the fungus <u>Blastomyces dermatitidis</u>, which is native to North America. Treatment with amphotericin B has been employed.

Aspergillosis is a relatively rare infection in AIDS patients (2). It may cause skin lesions, attack the lungs, or cause damage to the central nervous system. Amphotericin B has been used to treat this disease.

<u>Bacterial</u> Infections - <u>Shigellosis</u>, <u>Salmonellosis</u> & <u>Nacardiosis</u>

Shigellosis, caused by the bacteria <u>Shigella flexneri</u>, causes a severe diarrhea which may continue for months if not treated. This agent is often responsible for the rapid weight loss commonly seen in those having AIDS. However, it is not the only possible cause of diarrhea as <u>Salmonella enteritidis</u>, <u>Cryptosporidium difficile</u>, and cytomegalovirus may also cause diarrheas in individuals with AIDS (19).

Treatment of shigellosis has been undertaken with the drugs ampicillin, tetracycline, and trimethoprim sulfamethoxazole. After the initial infection, continual treatment may be necessary to prevent reoccurrence (17). When shigellosis and cytomegalovirus occur together, both diseases must be treated for a successful outcome. Colonoscopy is recommended as a means of confirming the presence of both types of infection (19).

<u>Salmonella enteritidis</u>, the agent that causes salmonellosis, is a difficult bacteria to to defeat. It may

cause digestive discomfort, bacterial infections, lesions in the brain, and attack the bone marrow. Drugs used to treat salmonella are ampicillin, amoxicillin, and tri-methoprim sulfamethoxazole with a prolonged treatment being necessary to keep the disease from recurring (17).

Nocardiosis, caused by <u>Nocardia</u> <u>asteroides</u>, may result in lesions on the skin or lungs, brain abscesses, and some forms of tumors, particularly on the feet. The administration of sulfadiazine on a daily basis for seve-ral months is a traditional treatment (Taber, 1981).

<u>Virus</u> <u>Infections</u> - <u>Cytomegalovirus</u>, <u>Herpes</u> <u>simplex</u>, & <u>Papovavirus</u>

Cytomegalovirus, frequently referred to as a CMV infection, is the most deadly viral infection associated with AIDS. It causes pneumonia, a discoloration and clouding of the retina of the eye (retinitis), and may also involve the intestinal tract and breathing passages (20). The retinitis may lead to blindness in one or both eyes, although some restoration of vision may result if damage to the eye is not too severe.

DPHG (9-(1,3 dihydroxy-2-propoxymethyl) guanine), a new drug related to acyclovir, has been successfully used to reduce the level of virus activity in the body and has partly restored vision loss caused by retinitis as well as clinical improvements in other CMV-related diseases in a group of 14 test patients at Mt. Zion Hospital in San Francisco (20).

Foscarnet (trisodium phosphonoformate) has been used by P. Christophe in limited human trials at the Claude Bernard Hospital in Paris with resulting clinical im-provements (35). More trials of this drug are now in progress. Relapses following withdrawal of the drug were noted, and maintenance therapy appears necessary with CMV-related diseases as it is with most, if not all, AIDS-associated opportunistic infections to prevent their reappearance.

Infection with the Herpes simplex virus is generally more severe in AIDS patients than in the normal population. There may be a large area of the body with numerous blister-like eruptions; the lungs may be infected, leading to pneumonia, and the virus may enter the brain and spinal cord, causing encephalitis. Viral infections are difficult to treat. Ara-A has been used with some success on herpes infections, and acyclovir may be useful in its treatment (Cuff, 1984).

Papoviruses are a group of viruses associated with cancers and, particularly in the case of AIDS, with multifocal lesions of the brain.

Cancer - Lymphoma of the Brain

This particular cancer is located in that part of the lymphatic system that services the brain. Typically this cancer is not localized, but located at many sites within the brain.

AIDS-RELATED COMPLEX (ARC)

The term, "AIDS-related complex" or ARC, is used to describe a series of symptoms thought to be related to infection with the HTLV-III virus, but which does not represent the severe end of the clinical spectrum required for the official definition of AIDS. Some have termed these symptoms "Pre-AIDS," but this usage is being discontinued because there is not sufficient evidence to demonstrate that ARC will lead inevitably into full-blown AIDS. However, a person with ARC has a higher probability of developing AIDS than a one who is symptom free. An Orange County, California, clinic reports that nearly 20 percent of ARC patients progressed to AIDS within 15 months after the diagnosis of ARC (which also means that 80 percent of their patients still did not have AIDS more than a year after the diagnosis of ARC) (Peskin, 1984).

According to the CDC, a person officially diagnosed as having ARC must have two clinical and two positive laboratory tests. The clinical symptoms, which must have persisted for three months or more with no other identifiable cause, include: fever of more than 100 degrees, diarrhea, night sweats, fatigue, weight loss of 10 percent of former body weight or more than 15 pounds without a change in diet or exercise habits, and a markedly reduced white blood cell count (1).

Of least two of the following laboratory tests must indicate: depressed helper T-cell numbers, a depressed helper to suppressor T-cell ratio, elevated serum globulin, depressed response to pokeweed and PRA antigens, the inability to respond normally to a variety of skin tests and have either leukopenia, thrombocytopenia, absolute lymphopenia or anemia (the latter series being a serious reduction of different types of blood cells). Notably absent in these tests is any reference to the detection of the AIDS virus or being in a risk group.

Psychological symptoms which have been reported in ARC patients include forgetfulness, memory loss, inability to concentrate, decreased hand-eye coordination, malaise, personality change, and changes in work and recreational habits. These symptoms apparently become more obvious as the disease progresses (21).

Because of relatively limited investigations of psychological disorders in AIDS patients, it is difficult to determine which symptoms are a result of the diagnosis of ARC or AIDS and which reflect an organic disorder. The first four symptoms listed in the previous paragraph relate to neurological function, whereas the remaining three can relate either to neurological disfunction or to the trauma of facing the realization that one has a potentially fatal disease.

PEDIATRIC AIDS

The establishment of new guidelines for the determination of the presence of AIDS in children was proposed at the International Conference on AIDS held in Atlanta in 1985. The reasons cited for the need for such a definition included the facts that the young may not necessarily exhibit the range of symptoms required by the present definition, even though they may succumb to the disease. This is particularly true of children infected at birth (22).

The CDC published a provisional case definition for AIDS in children in December of 1983 which is reproduced below:

PROVISIONAL CASE DEFINITION FOR ACQUIRED IMMUNODEFICIENCY SYNDROME (AIDS) IN CHILDREN (23).

For the limited purposes of epidemiologic surveillance, CDC defines a case of pediatric-acquired immunodeficiency syndrome (AIDS) as a child who has had:

1. a reliably diagnosed disease at least moderately indicative of underlying cellular immunodeficiency and

2. no known cause of underlying cellular immunodeficiency or any other reduced resistance reported to be associated with that disease.

The diseases accepted as sufficiently indicative of underlying cellular immunodeficiency are the same as those used in defining AIDS in adults with the exclusion of congenital infections; e.g., toxoplasmosis or herpes simplex virus infection in the first month after birth or cytomegalovirus infection in the first 6 months after birth.

Specific conditions that must be excluded in a child are:

1. Primary immunodeficiency diseases -- severe combined immunodeficiency: DiGeorge syndrome, Wiskott-Aldrich syndrome, ataxia-telangiectasia, graft versus host disease, neutropenia, neutrophil function abnormality, gammaglobulinemia, or hypogammaglobulinemia with raised igM.

2. Secondary immunodeficiency associated with immunosuppressive therapy, lymphoreticular malignancy, or starvation.

The present CDC definition of AIDS in children is practically identical to that used to define AIDS in adults with the exception of the exclusionary factors.

Children with AIDS have a high mortality rate with one study reporting a 40 percent mortality rate among 34 pediatric patients (24). With aggressive treatment starting with diet, rapid therapy to defeat infections, correction of anemia, and IV gammaglobulin treatment, clinical improvement was seen in patients receiving the IV gammaglobulin infusions (24).

GERIATRIC AIDS

Geriatric AIDS is a potential problem that has not been specifically dealt with at the international conferences on AIDS, and little literature has been produced on this subject. Although a geriatric is somewhat less likely to contract AIDS by sexual contact with an infected individual, the risk of contracting AIDS during a blood transfusion administered during a past surgery would appear to be somewhat greater in the older segment of the population. There is a risk that the onset of AIDS might be masked by preexisting diseases, like emphysema, and the patient die from AIDS without its ever being diagnosed.

CONCLUSIONS

AIDS is a devastating syndrome marked by a variety of possible manifestations with the potential of serially or simultaneously affecting virtually every organ of the body with one or more different diseases. With the present state of knowledge, the survival of a person with AIDS for a period longer than five years after the diagnosis of AIDS is not very favorable. Deterioration and death can occur quite rapidly, depending on the type of AIDS-associated disease that the patient contracts, although with existing treatment some opportunistic diseases can be defeated for years.

Rapid progress is being made to more successfully treat the AIDS-associated diseases as well as to kill or neutralize the AIDS virus itself. If a technique can be found to rid the body of the AIDS virus and restore some of the damage done to the body's immune system, there is a real possibility that even seriously ill AIDS patients could be helped.

---

1. Centers For Disease Control, 1984, The case definition of AIDS used by CDC for epidemiologic Surveillance: Atlanta, Georgia, May.

2. Armstrong, Donald A., 1985, Management of infection in AIDS patients: Memorial Sloan-Kettering Cancer Center, New York, International Conference on AIDS, Atlanta, Georgia.

3. Filson, C. Richard, 1985, Psychological characteristics of individuals with AIDS-related concerns: Georgetown University Medical Center, Washington D.C., International Conference on AIDS, Atlanta, Georgia.

4. Michael, Philip, 1985, Significance of persistence of P. carinii after completion of treatment: university of California, San Francisco, International Conference on AIDS, Atlanta, Georgia.

5. Garay, Stuart M., 1985, Pneumocystis carinii pneumonia in the acquired immunodeficiency syndrome: New York University Medical Center, New York, International Conference on AIDS, Atlanta, Georgia.

6. Hardy, David, 1985, Fansidar prophylaxis for Pneumocystis carinii Pneumonia: University of California, Los Angeles, International Conference on AIDS, Atlanta, Georgia.

7. Richardson, Susan, 1985, Diaminodiphenylsulfone (dapsone) as treatment for Pneumocystis carinii pneumonia in AIDS patients in combination with trimethoprim: University of Toronto, Canada, International Conference on AIDS, Atlanta, Georgia.

8. Hawkins, Catherine, 1985, Treatment of M. avium-intra-

cellularae infection in AIDS: Memorial Sloan-Kettering Cancer Center, New York, International Conference on AIDS, Atlanta, Georgia.

9. Good, Robert C., 1985, Bacteriology of mycobacterial isolates from patients with AIDS: Centers For Disease Control, Atlanta, Georgia, International Conference on AIDS, Atlanta, Georgia.

10. O'Brien, R.J., 1985, Anamycin LM427 therapy in AIDS patients with Mycobacterium avium complex infection; A Preliminary Report: Centers For Disease Control, Atlanta, Georgia, International Conference on AIDS, Atlanta Georgia.

11. Safai, Bijan, 1985, The natural history of Kaposi's sarcoma in individuals with AIDS: Memorial Sloan-Kettering Cancer Center, New York, International Conference on AIDS, Atlanta, Georgia.

12. Volderding, Paul A., 1985, Vinblastine therapy of AIDS-Related Kaposi's sarcoma: Anderson Hospital, Houston, Texas, International Conference on AIDS, Atlanta, Georgia.

13. Rios, Adan, 1985, The Use of interferon in the treatment of acquired immunodeficiency syndrome-related Kaposi's sarcoma: Anderson, Hospital, Houston, Texas, International Conference on AIDS, Atlanta, Georgia.

14. Ungar, Beth L.P.,1985, Serologic response to Cryptosporidium detected by enzyme-linked immunosorbent assay (ELISA): Cornell University Medical Center, New York and Animal Parasitology Institute, Beltsville, Maryland, International Conference on AIDS, Atlanta, Georgia.

15. Price, Richard W., 1985, Neurological complications of AIDS; An overview based on 110 autopsied patients: Cornell University Medical Center, New York; Medical College of New Jersey, Newark; and Memorial Sloan-Kettering Cancer Center, New York, International Conference on AIDS, Atlanta, Georgia.

16. Lunde, Milford N., 1985, Diagnostic studies for toxoplasmosis in AIDS: National Institutes of

Health, Bethesda, Maryland, and George Washington University, Washington D.C., International
Conference on AIDS, Atlanta, Georgia.

17. Whimbey, Estella, 1985, Bacteremia and fungemia in
patients with AIDS: Memorial Sloan-Kettering
Cancer Center, New York, International Conference on AIDS, Atlanta, Georgia.

18. Small, Catherine B., 1985, The acquired immunodeficiency syndrome and disseminated histoplasmosis
in a nonendemic area: New York Medical College,
Valhalla; Misericordia Hospital and Medical
Center, Bronx; Metropolitan Hospital, New York;
and Westchester County Medical Center, Valhalla, New York, International Conference on AIDS,
Atlanta, Georgia.

19. Bell, Evan T., 1985, Simultaneous shigellosis and cytomegalovirus colitis in patients with acquired
immunodeficiency syndrome: Lenox Hill Hospital,
New York, International Conference on AIDS,
Atlanta, Georgia.

20. Drew, W.L., 1985, Evaluation of DHPG against cytomegalovirus infection in AIDS patients: Mt. Zion
Hospital., Ralph K. Davies Medical Center, St.
Luke's Hospital., and the University of California, San Francisco, International Conference
on AIDS, Atlanta, Georgia.

21. Tross, Susan, 1985, Psychological and neuropsycholog-
ical function in AIDS spectrum disorder patients: Memorial Sloan-Kettering Cancer Center
and Cornell University Medical College, New
York, International Conference on AIDS, Atlanta, Georgia.

22. Ammann, Arthur, 1985, Defining AIDS in children: U-
niversity of California Medical Center, San
Francisco, International Conference on AIDS,
Atlanta, Georgia.

23. Centers for Disease Control, 1984, Update; acquired
immunodeficiency syndrome (AIDS) -- United
States: Centers for Disease Control, Atlanta,
Georgia, January 6.

24. Oleske, James, 1985, Therapy of pediatric-acquired immune deficiency syndrome, poster W-21, International Conference on AIDS, Atlanta, Georgia.

25. Centers for Disease Control, 1986, Classification system for human T-lymphotropic virus Type III/lymphadenopathy-associated virus infections: Mortality Weekly Report, May 23.

26. Redfield, Robert, R., 1986, The natural history of HTLV-III/LAV infection: Walter Reed Army Inst. of Research and Walter Reed Army Medical Center, Second International Conference on AIDS, Paris, France.

27. Barlow, J.L.R., 1986, Treatment of Pneumocystis carinii pneumonia with eflornithine: Second International Conference on AIDS, Paris, France.

28. Rozenbaum, W., 1986, Treatment of AIDS-related infections: Dept. Sante Publique et Maladies Infectieuses, Hopital Pitie-Salpetriere, Paris, Second International Conference on AIDS, Paris, France.

29. Inderlied, C.B., 1986, Mycobacterium avium complex (MAC) from AIDS patients: antimicrobial susceptibility and evaluation of potential treatment regimens in an animal model of disseminated MAC infection: Kuzell Institute, Pacific Presbyterian Medical Center, San Francisco, California, Second International Conference on AIDS, Paris, France.

30. Rozenbaum, W., 1986, Treatment of AIDS-related Kaposi's sarcoma by alpha-2 recombinant interferon: Dept. of Public Health and Tropical Medicine Pitie-Salpetriere Hospital, Paris, Second International Conference on AIDS, Paris, France.

31. Miles, Steven A., 1986, Phase I trial of recombinant interferon Gamma in AIDS-related Kaposi's Sarcoma (AIDS/KS): UCLA School of Medicine, Los Angeles, Second International Conference on AIDS, Paris, France.

32. Centers for Disease Control, 1984, Update: treatment of cryptosporidiosis in patients with acquired

immunodeficiency syndrome (AIDS): Mortality Weekly Report, March 9.

33. Raffi, F., 1986, Treatment of brain toxoplasmosis with pyrimethamine and sulfadiazine in 35 AIDS patients: efficacy of long-term continuous therapy: Hopital Claude Bernard, Paris, Second International Conference on AIDS, Paris, France.

34. Centers for Disease Control, 1986, Recommended infection control practices for dentistry: Mortality Weekly Report, April 18.

35. Christophe, P., 1986, Foscarnet for cytomegalovirus (CMV) infections in AIDS: Hopital Claude Bernard, Paris, Second International Conference on AIDS, Paris, France.

Peskind, Steve, 1984, Living with AIDS; an information guide for Orange County (Calif.): AIDS Response Program of Orange County and the University of California Irvine Medical Center, Garden Grove, California, 109 p.

Cuff, Mary, 1984, New York University Hospital (in above p.16-17).

Taber, Clarence Wilber, 1983, Taber's cyclopedic medical dictionary, 14th edition: F.A. Davis Co., Philadelphia, Pennsylvania, 1818 p.

THE AIDS EPIDEMIC

TO THOSE WHO HAVE AIDS, 1981 seems a long time ago; and recalling what life was like before the AIDS epidemic is similar to remembering how life was in the United States before Vietnam. Because of AIDS, life in America is different and will never be the same again. In the late 1970s and early 1980s the gay liberation movement was asserting its power with a new emphasis on gay pride. The result was that many gays who had led closeted sex lives were moving to metropolitan centers where there was freedom to practice their life styles without the social stigmatization common in other parts of the country.

In New York, San Francisco, and Los Angeles, gays were active in all professions and not restricted to those related to the arts, health care, or interior decorating where popular stereotypes placed them. One release by the CDC in June of 1982 estimated that there were between 185,000 to 415,000 gay males living in Los Angeles County, about 8 percent of the county's adult male population, who were exclusively homosexual and 18 percent who were bisexual.

A December, 1984, survey from San Francisco reported that there were some 70,000 gay men in the city, or nearly 10 percent of the population of about 707,000. This study estimated that 45,000 gays immigrated into the city between 1974 and 1985. In terms of age, two-thirds of the total gay population were less than 39 (1).

As New York and San Francisco began to be known as "Gay Capitals," they attracted business that catered to the social and sexual activities of a group of gay men and women who were dominantly between the ages of 18 and 45. Bath houses, gay bars, gay movie houses, gay hotels, and other establishments that were limited only by the imagination of their owners flourished to satisfy the interest and appetites of a prosperous gay population.

Also attracted to these cities were numbers of teen runaways who prostituted themselves to gays in order to earn a living. This condition was also found in Haiti, where boys engaged in prostitution to earn a livelihood and later resumed a heterosexual sex life (2).

With these inducements, gays from other parts of the country went to the larger cities for "Sex Vacations" and, if their finances allowed, also visited European cities like Amsterdam which had reputations of being "Gay Capitols" of Europe. Europeans likewise came to the United States seeking gay sex and found it to be abundantly available in the larger cities (3).

The number of penetrative encounters occurring among gays during a single night in a city like New York could easily rank on the order of hundreds a night. Some homosexual males in later follow-up studies reported up to 200 sexual contacts per year (4).

These factors provided a pool of individuals whose life styles had a high risk for the contraction and transmission of venereal diseases. This fact was recognized by public health providers in cities with large gay populations, and clinics were established in which to treat sexually-transmitted diseases (STDs) along with providing community health care.

Although no one knew it at the time, the mechanisms had been established whereby a disease with a long incubation period would be rapidly transmitted worldwide. For two years or more the gay community unknowingly infected each other and their heterosexual partners with the most devastating sexually transmitted disease that the world has seen.

In addition to sexual contact, blood donations by infected individuals provided a means of transmitting AIDS to receivers of blood and blood products in the United States and also to European and Asian countries which imported American blood products.

At some early stage, and it is futile to speculate precisely when this occurred, drug users became infected with AIDS. Users of intravenous (IV) drugs transmitted the disease among themselves, to their sexual partners, and to some of their subsequent children. AIDS among drug users was, and remains, more prevalent near large cities where the availability of drugs is high.

A NEW VENEREAL SYNDROME

By 1981 when the first five cases of Pneumocystis carinii pneumonia in gay men were reported from Los Angeles, the AIDS virus was already being disseminated through the United States, Africa, Europe, and Australia by sexual contact, contaminated blood products, and illegal IV drug use (5). Blind chance had created the optimum conditions for the AIDS epidemic.

The weekly Morbidity and Mortality Report issued by the Centers for Disease Control reported in June, 1981, the occurrence of the five cases of Pneumocystis carinii pneumonia between October, 1980, and May of 1981. The report stated, "The fact that these patients were all homosexuals suggests an association between some aspect of a homosexual lifestyle or disease acquired through sexual contact and Pneumocystis pneumonia in this population (5)." This suggested association proved to be true and was reinforced as more cases of PCP as well as Kaposi's sarcoma and other immune suppression-related diseases were reported to the CDC.

The name, Acquired Immune Deficiency Syndrome (AIDS), first appeared in a CDC report dated September 24, 1982, in which the following tables appeared (6). Most of the cases reported in 1979 and some of those from 1980 were determined retrospectively. The earliest cases of AIDS that could be recognized from the symptomatology appeared in New York City as early as the mid-1970's (7).

The word "epidemic" was not used in the conservative language of the official CDC report, but the figures in the two tables revealed in a dramatic fashion the mortality of the disease and its apparent rapid spread throughout the United States. This report, perhaps more than any other document, made it abundantly clear that a serious new sexually transmitted disease was infecting primarily

Table 2. Reported cases and mortality rates of AIDS, by half-year of diagnosis 1979-1982, (as of September 15, 1982) - U. S.

Half-year of diagnosis		Cases	Deaths	Percent mortality
1979	1st half	1	1	100
	2nd half	6	5	83
1980	1st half	17	13	76
	2nd half	26	22	85
1981	1st half	66	46	70
	2nd half	141	79	56
1982	1st half	249	67	27

Table 3. AIDS cases per million population, by standard metropolitan statistical area (SMSA) of residence, reported from June 1, 1981, to September 15, 1982 - U.S.

Residence	Cases	Percentage of total	Cases per million
New York	288	48.6	31.6
San Francisco	78	13.2	24.0
Miami	31	5.2	19.1
Newark	15	2.5	7.6
Houston	15	6.2	4.9
Elsewhere	129	21.9	0.6

gay men, but also intravenous drug abusers, Haitians (since discounted as an ethnic risk group (8)), and perhaps hemophiliacs.

Something was known of how and how rapidly the disease was spreading and of the mortality of the disease, but little else. Not until November 5, 1982, did the CDC speculate that, "One hypothesis consistent with current observations is that a transmissible agent may be involved. If so, transmission of the agent would appear most commonly to require intimate direct contact involving mucosal surfaces, such as sexual contact among homosexual males, or through parenteral spread such as occurs among intravenous drug abusers and possibly hemophilia patients using Factor VIII products (to prevent bleeding episodes) (9)." The same release stated, "These patterns resemble the distribution of disease and modes of spread of hepatitis B virus, and hepatitis B virus infections occur very frequently among AIDS patients."

By December 10, 1982, the link had been made between AIDS and hemophilia A patients who received Factor VIII blood concentrates suspected to be contaminated with some AIDS-causing agent (10). In addition, an infant was documented as contracting AIDS after receiving blood from a donor who later died as a result of AIDS-related diseases. This evidence further indicated that the AIDS-causing agent was an infectious agent capable of being transferred from person-to-person by sexual intercourse and by blood or blood products.

A month later the CDC issued a release warning that female sexual partners of AIDS patients were at risk of contracting AIDS by documenting two cases of women with no other risk factors who apparently contracted AIDS from their sex partners. Although not heralded as such at the time, this January 7, 1983, release marked the first time AIDS had been found to have spread outside closely defined risk groups into the general heterosexual population (11).

Say, for example, that a heterosexual man had sex with someone in New York in 1983. If his one-time partner had AIDS and the man contracted the virus, that man could be symptom-free for perhaps eight years or longer before the onset of disease. In the meantime, even if the man had been faithful to his wife, except for that one episode, he could have infected his wife with the result that she and any subsequent children would have a high risk of developing AIDS.

Women prostitutes in larger cities like New York, San Francisco, and Miami also fell under suspicion as possible transmitters of AIDS. But since there was no easily-applied test for the syndrome until 1985, there was no means of proving transmission via women prostitutes until they had been linked by contact tracing to a person who had developed AIDS.

The following list of recommendations for avoiding AIDS was published by the CDC in March, 1983 (12).

1. Sexual contact should be avoided with persons known or suspected to have AIDS. Members of high risk groups (and now everyone) should be aware that multiple sexual partners increase the probability of developing AIDS.

2. As a temporary measure, members of groups at increased risk for AIDS should refrain from donating plasma and/or blood, even though many individuals are at little risk of AIDS. Centers collecting plasma and/or blood should inform potential donors of this recommendation. The Food and Drug Administration is preparing new recommendations for manufacturers of plasma derivative and for establishments collecting plasma or blood. This is an interim measure to protect recipients of blood products and blood until specific laboratory tests are available.

3. Studies should be conducted to evaluate screening procedures for their effectiveness in identifying and excluding plasma and blood with a high probability of transmitting AIDS. These procedures should include specific laboratory tests as well as careful histories and physical examinations.

4. Physicians should adhere strictly to medical indications for transfusions and autologous blood transfusions (using a patient's own blood collected prior to surgery) are encouraged.

5. Work should continue toward development of safer

blood products for use by hemophilia patients.

There could be little practical expectation that the guidelines would have any short-term effect on the spread of AIDS because of its long incubation period. In September, 1983, a year after the information on Tables 2 and 3 had been compiled, there were 2,259 reported cases of AIDS in the United States compared with a total of 506 cases reported between 1979 and September of 1983 -- a four-fold increase (13). Cases that had been infected months or years prior to publication of the guidelines were progressing into full-blown disease.

The Virus Identified

By May of 1983, Luc Montagnier of the Pasteur Institute in Paris published that the institute had identified a lymphadenopathy-associated virus, LAV, that was responsible for AIDS. The virus had been first isolated from a lymph node of a New York man, and later the same virus was found in patients from Central Africa. A series of 30 test samples was sent to the institute by the CDC. Ten of these samples were from uninfected men, with equal numbers of samples from ARC and AIDS patients. The institute successfully identified each of these samples, finding the AIDS virus in all 20 of the samples from ARC and AIDS patients (14).

In the meantime, the search for the virus was also

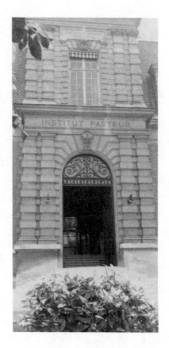

Figure 5. Pasteur Institute, Paris.

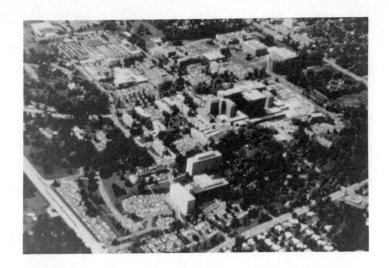

Figure 6. The National Institutes of Health at Bethesda,
Maryland, where, at the National Cancer Institute,
Robert C. Gallo cultured the virus which he named
the HTLV-III (AIDS) virus. This discovery was announced in April, 1984, 13 months after the LAV
virus was described by Luc Montagnier and others at
the Pasteur Institute in Paris. Although yet a
third AIDS-causing virus, ARV, has also been announced by Jay Levy from the University of California at San Francisco, all three are considered variations of the same virus. NIH photo.

underway in the United States. Approximately a year
after the French discovery of LAV, Margaret Heckler, then
secretary of the United States Department of Health and
Human Services, announced in April, 1984, the discovery
of the HTLV-III (AIDS) virus by Robert C. Gallo and
others at the National Cancer Institute (14).

In addition, Jay Levy at the University of California at San Francisco identified what he termed AIDS-
related virus, ARV (14). Most researchers, while a-
greeing that there are differences between the viruses
identified as LAV, HTLV-III, and ARV, view these virus

strains as the same AIDS-causing agent. This is something like recognizing that German shepherds, French poodles, and the Mexican hairless are all dogs, even though they differ in appearance.

Gallo, speaking at the First International Conference on AIDS, stated while he thought that competition between labs was desirable when it became nationalistic it was, "science debased and ought to be rooted out like the weed that it is (15)," and Montagnier agreed (3).

The AIDS virus, previously known as HTLV-III/LAV, was renamed HIV, Human Immunodeficiency Virus, in 1986 by the International Committee for the Taxonomy of Viruses as reported by the CDC in the July 4, 1986, issue of the Mortality Weekly Report.

While the new name should help avoid confusion among the three names already introduced for the virus, HTLV-III, LAV, and ARV, it has not been universally adopted. The CDC, for example, still uses the name HTLV-III/LAV, as does much current literature. In time, the name HIV will be commonly used, as it was by many presenters at the Second International Conference On AIDS in 1986. Gallo, in commenting on the new name, stated that he had no objection to the use of HIV other than the reservation that any virus products sent from the National Institutes of Health continue to be identified by their original name so as to leave no doubt as to what particular variant of the virus was being used (22).

World Prevalence of AIDS

At the 1985 international conference, Jean-Baptiste Brunet of the World Health Organization reported that AIDS occurred on five continents, North and South America, Europe, Africa, and Australia. In the Americas, AIDS had been reported in the United States (8,397 cases), Canada (165 cases), Brazil (182 cases), and Haiti (340 cases), as well as in 11 other countries with from one to 16 cases each. Haiti had the highest rate of infection with 59.6 cases per million inhabitants compared to the

TABLE 4. World prevalence of AIDS, May 21, 1986, World
Health Organization.*

Continent	No. Cases	No. of Countries
Africa	378	9
Americas	22,085	43
Asia	50	11
Europe	2,423	27
Oceania	214	2
Total	25,150	92

Note: This table represents officially reported cases in
countries which report to WHO. It was admitted by
officials of WHO that these figures, particularly for
Africa, were unrealistically low estimates.

United States with 35.8 cases per million (17).

Speaking a year later at the second international
conference, H. Mahler of the World Health Organization
(WHO) stated that over 20,000 cases had been reported to
that organization since 1981 with over 75 percent of that
number reported in 1984 and 1985. He said that most of
these cases, 85 percent, were from the United States and
expressed concern about apparently large, but incompletely reported, number of AIDS cases in over 20 African
countries. He said that his best estimate of the world-
wide prevalence of AIDS was that from 5-10 million individuals were infected with the AIDS virus, and the total
number of AIDS cases were between 30-50,000 (22).

Europe, with a reported 2,542 cases (updated information given during oral presentation), falls behind
North America in the number of cases, but some countries
report a rate of development of new AIDS cases equivalent
to rate of increase in the United States. In France, for
example, there is a doubling of the number of cases
approximately every eight months or a rate of increase of

163 percent per year (23).

Relatively few cases are reported from Asia, but AIDS cases or virus-positive tests are seen in Thailand, Hong Kong, Vietnam, and the U.S.S.R. (24, 25, 26). These Asian cases, and the similar low incidences of cases in some Central and South American countries, do not indicate any natural resistance to AIDS, but only that the disease was introduced later than in Africa and North America. Asia and South America contain much of the world's population, and there is hope that an aggressive educational program can prevent the explosive spread of AIDS on these continents.

AIDS in Europe

AIDS is also viewed with alarm in Europe. The CDC reported figures from the World Health Organization Collaborating Center on Acquired Immunodeficiency Syndrome in Paris that there were 421 cases of AIDS on the conti-

Table 5. Reported AIDS cases -- 10 European countries as of July 15, 1984.

Country	Cases	Per million population
Denmark	28	5.5
France	180	3.4
West Germany	79	1.3
Greece	2	0.2
Italy	8	0.1
Netherlands	21	1.5
Spain	14	0.4
Sweden	7	0.8
Switzerland	28	4.4
United Kingdom	54	1.0
Total	421	

Centers for Disease Control

nent as of July, 1984 (16) (see Table 5).

Eight months later, a January 18, 1985, release by the CDC reported that there were 559 cases of AIDS in 12 European countries with about 10 new cases being diagnosed each week (18).

Table 6. Reported AIDS cases -- 15 European countries as of January 18, 1985

Country	Cases	Per million population
Denmark	31	6.0
Finland	4	0.8
France	221	4.0
West Germany	110	1.8
Greece	2	0.2
Italy	10	0.2
Netherlands	26	1.8
Norway	4	1.0
Spain	18	0.5
Sweden	12	1.5
Switzerland	33	5.0
United Kingdom	88	1.6
Total	559	

Centers for Disease Control

In Europe, 17 countries in 1985 reported AIDS data with the highest rates of infection in Denmark, Switzerland, France, and Belgium. (The reason that Belgium is not reported in tables 5 and 6 is unknown.) (17). The incidence rates reported from Paris and Geneva are now comparable to the rates observed in Los Angeles. AIDS arrived at different times in various European countries between 1981 and 1983. The difference in incidence rates in the various countries mostly depends on the time that the disease has been present (17).

By the time of the second international conference in 1986, European nations reporting to the WHO listed

Table 7. Reported AIDS cases -- 21 European countries as of September 30, 1985

Country	Cases	Per million population
Austria	23	3.1
Belgium	118	11.9
Denmark	57	11.2
Federal Republic of Germany	295	4.8
Finland	10	2.0
France	466	8.5
Greece	10	1.0
Italy	92	1.6
Luxembourg	3	7.5
Netherlands	83	5.7
Norway	14	3.3
Spain	63	1.6
Sweden	36	4.3
Switzerland	77	11.8
United Kingdom	225	4.0
Yugoslavia	1	0.0
Total	1,573	

Centers for Disease Control

2,542 cases. France again led Europe with the largest number of cases, 707 (221 in 1985) the Federal Republic of Germany followed with 457 (110 in 1985) with the third highest number of cases being from the United Kingdom, 340 (88 in 1985). Countries listed with the highest rates of infection were Belgium, Switzerland and Denmark (22).

Differences of prevalence of routes of infectivity had also become apparent by 1986 with J-B. Brunet of WHO reporting that in northern European countries homosexuals accounted for 80 percent of AIDS cases, whereas in southern Europe IV drug users accounted for the highest percentage, 50 percent, of the cases (27).

All of the 27 hemophiliac cases of AIDS in Europe documented in 1985 were from countries that imported blood products from the United States, such as Belgium, France, and Denmark. Those countries that utilized their own blood products (principally the Factor VIII to promote blood clotting) reported no cases of AIDS in hemophiliacs treated with their products (17), and all European are now screening blood donations for the AIDS virus.

Sexual tourism, AIDS-contaminated blood products, and immigration by natives and former residents of Central Africa were cited as being the principal means by which AIDS was introduced into Europe (17).

AIDS in Africa

Several lines of evidence point to Central Africa as the place of origin for the AIDS virus (15). AIDS had been reported in 18 different countries (17) including Zaire, Congo, Gabon, Mali, Zambia, Cameroon, Cape Verde, Ghana, Togo, Rwanda, Burundi, Tanzania, Kenya, and Uganda in 1985 and had by 1986 been also identified in Senegal, South Africa, and Malawi. In Uganda, 65 percent of school children who had blood drawn in 1972 were later found to give positive tests for AIDS antibodies (15).

Information presented at the Second International Conference on AIDS indicated that some of the original high prevalence figures, such as the test on school children's blood in Uganda, were suspect because of inconsistencies in testing techniques.

In summarizing more recent, more reliable, testing, B.M. Kapita from the Mama Yemo Hospital in Kinshasa, Zaire, stated that the prevalence rate of AIDS infection was as high as 80 percent in some high risk groups (particularly prostitutes) in Central and East Africa, 6 percent in Southern Africa, and 14 percent from the rest of the continent (28). He also cited seroprevalence figures of 0-24 percent from Southern Africa (South Africa and Malawi), 4-6 percent from Central Africa (Central Af-

Arican Republic and Zaire) and West Africa (Senegal), and of 18-23 percent seropositivity from East Africa (Rwanda and Uganda).

At present the number of cases on the African continent are estimated to be on the order of 50,000 cases of AIDS with approximately 2 million infected with the virus. Because of incomplete reporting, Kapita stated that the 378 officially reported cases were far short of representing the prevalence of the disease in Africa (28).

All workers reporting data from Africa stated that sexual contact was the most important factor in the rapid spread of AIDS on the continent. Prostitutes were cited by many as being a significant factor in the spread of the syndrome.

In a study of prostitutes in Kinshasa, Zaire, J.M. Mann reported that out of 357 female prostitutes, 27 percent tested positively for AIDS antibodies. He also reported that the group reported an average of 3.7 sexual partners a week, 158 a year, and 703 lifetime sexual partners (29).

The heterosexual spread of AIDS in Africa was documented by P. Piot. This author gave evidence that there were equal numbers of male to female cases; there was a promiscuous heterosexual lifestyle among many patients, a high percentage of female prostitutes and "free women" among AIDS cases, clusters of AIDS cases linked by heterosexual contact, and a high seropositivity rate in heterosexual partners of infected individuals (30).

J. Desmyter examined blood samples taken during 1970 from 805 healthy mothers from Kinshasa, Zaire, and compared this data with results obtained from a sample of 498 healthy mothers in 1980. He found that 17 samples from 1970 tested positively for the virus and 22 tested positively from 1980. This result, about a 10-fold increase in 10 years, compared with the expected 500-fold increase in cases in the United States among homosexuals and drug users, demonstrated that heterosexual activity was a less efficient way to transmit the virus, but still represented a serious health risk (31).

A new virus, LAV 2, also known as HTLV-IV, has been confirmed by both the Pasteur Institutes and the National Institutes of Health from blood taken from West Africans with AIDS. F. Clavel summarized the findings on this virus as, "These findings indicate that LAV-II is a novel (new) retrovirus related to, but distinct from, LAV and HTLV-III (32)." The new virus may not attack T-4 cells, and its possible pathologic effects are uncertain. It is known that HTLV-IV does not give a positive result with present ELISA test designed to detect antibodies to the HTLV-III/LAV (HIV) virus.

Another French worker from the institute, Marc Alizon, reported that the AIDS virus was present in Zaire before the onset of AIDS cases in the United States and Europe and pointed out the similarities of this virus and a simian-AIDS virus cultured from wild African monkeys. He suggested that the two viruses may share a common origin derived from the mutation of a parent retrovirus (33). The genetic characteristics of HTLV-IV indicate that it may be an even closer relative of the simian-AIDS virus than HTLV-III/LAV (HIV).

Recognition of the Danger

The gay population of the United States, who were by 1984 largely informed of the risk of AIDS by the gay press and popular media, began changing their social habits. A telling warning to gays was when the word circulated that Jack or Tom or Louise or Paul, a person known to members of the community, was dying of AIDS. This news moved the personal realization of the syndrome to the point that, "Someone I know is dying with this stuff, and I could get it too. Maybe I already have it."

Some gays opted to refrain from sex until the AIDS crisis was over. Others entered monogamous relationships, with or without penetrative sex. More resolved to decrease the frequency of their sexual activity and/or refrain from penetrative sex while some opted to follow one or more of the "Safer Sex" guidelines issued by gay organizations or public health clinics. Human beings being what they are, a portion managed to keep their resolves; but others, at least occasionally, backslid into their pleasurable, but dangerous, old sex habits.

Nonetheless, the end result was a dramatic decrease in the sexual activities of gays. A CDC report in June, 1984, documented a decrease in the incidence of rectal gonorrhea among gay men at one New York clinic from 485 cases per 100,000 in 1980 to 201 per 100,000 in 1983. Among women visiting the clinic, the rates of rectal gonorrhea increased during the same period from 587 per 100,000 to 624 per 100,000 (19).

James W. Curran, of the CDC, stated at 1985 International Conference on AIDS that gay men all over the world had been reducing their numbers of sexual partners in what he termed was the most dramatic sexual revolution since the 1960s (20). He cited a San Francisco Health Department study which saw the incidence of rectal gonorrhea reduced from 5,000 cases in 1980 to just over 1,300 in 1984 -- a 73 percent decrease. This suggests gays have greatly reduced the number of sexual partners, but unfortunately the prevalence of the AIDS virus has increased, from 24 percent in 1980 to 68 percent in 1984 -- a nearly 200 percent increase (20).

A gay man in San Francisco with 12 sexual partners in 1980 would have been exposed to three potentially infectious men with positive AIDS antibody status. Even though that man may have reduced his sexual partners to three in 1984, two of those men would still be infected (20). As a result, the man's risk of exposure would be diminished only slightly, despite a dramatic change in behavior.

The June CDC report cited above offered the hope that, "The substantial and persistent declines in gonorrhea among homosexual males in New York City suggest that prevention efforts have succeeded in reducing the incidence of this ... sexually transmitted infection. Further sustained efforts should help in reducing the incidence of AIDS among homosexual males (19)."

At the time of the April, 1985, International Conference on AIDS, Curran stated that the 9,600 cases of AIDS reported to that time were expected to double by 1986 to 18,000 to 19,000 cases (20). Factors he recognized as complicating the estimation of the total rate of new case development were that from 5 to 20 percent of AIDS cases developed symptoms between two-to-five years after infection, but over 50 percent remained without symptoms for longer periods (20).

The same author reported at the Paris conference in June of 1986 that there were approximately 15,000 cases of AIDS diagnosed in the United States. Curran cautiously attributed some of the 3,000 fewer cases than projected to the first indications that "safer sex" practices by the gay community were beginning to slow the rate of new infections. He cautioned that 75 percent of cases of AIDS that would be diagnosed in 1991, the 10th anniversary of the recognition of the first cases of AIDS in the United States, were probably infected before "safer sex" practices were generally used (34).

Using current rates of transmission and assuming the absence of a vaccine or cure, Curran projected that in 1991 there would be 74,000 cases of AIDS diagnosed that year in the United States, 174,000 hospital confinements because of AIDS, 54,000 deaths from AIDS, and an annual treatment cost of $8 billion, averaging about $46,000 per patient. By 1991, he estimated that the accumulated total of AIDS cases in the United States would be 270,000, of which 179,000 would have died (34).

Blood samples collected during a hepatitis B study among San Francisco gay men between 1978 and 1980 were reanalyzed, and ten percent of the group participating in the original study were invited to participate in a new AIDS study to determine the rate of infection and the time between infection (indicated by the presence of the virus) and the onset of symptoms. The time between detection of the virus in blood samples and AIDS developing in the group was between three to four years, and a substantial portion of the group was found to have been infected before 1981 (20).

"Most communities are late in recognizing the severity of the AIDS problem, and can deny it, until a
large number of individuals are infected with the virus,"
Curran said. Based on an estimate made from a study of
6,875 men, Curran said in 1986 that he guessed that
between 1,000,000 and 1,500,000 Americans were infected
with the AIDS virus, an increase of 500,000 over his 1985
estimate (34).

AIDS infection may be a persistent, perhaps even a
life-long, infection; but the transmissibility of AIDS
through sex or to newborns may be intermittent (20).

Where We Stand Now

Now, four months after the Second International
Conference on AIDS, the disease is continuing to spread
in the United States and its rate of increase is resulting in a doubling of cases every 11 months. The high
estimate of the number of individuals in the United
States infected with the AIDS virus is now said to be
about 2,000,000, a number without attribution currently
banded about in the nation's newspapers (21).

Statistics from the CDC as of January 13, 1986, show
that of 16,458 people in the United States who have
contracted AIDS, 65.3 percent are homosexual or bisexual
men (down from 72 percent the previous year), 25.1 percent are I.V. drug users (up from 17 percent), 0.8
percent are hemophiliacs, 1.6 percent contracted AIDS as
a result of transfusions with AIDS-contaminated blood,
7.1 percent contracted AIDS through unknown causes, and
heterosexual contact accounted for 1.1 percent of the
cases (35). Of the 12,932 cases reported by the CDC as
of August 1, 1985, 6,481 had died; and the mortality rate
remains at about 50 percent (22).

In the United States, the August, 1985, report
stated that New York City led the nation with a reported
3,993 cases of AIDS, San Francisco followed with 1,371
cases, Los Angeles with 1,020 cases, Miami with 425,
Newark with 299 and the remainder of the nation, 4,959

cases, mostly occurring in the larger metropolitan areas (22).

If any comfort can be gathered from these grim statistics, it is that the percentage of heterosexual infections that have been reported remains at about one percent (1.1) of AIDS cases after reaching that level in 1982. This may demonstrate that the spread of AIDS through the heterosexual portion of the nation's population may be slower than is occurring among homosexuals and bisexuals as Curran (20) suggested, although approximately 4,000 adults in the United States professing exclusive heterosexuality have been infected with AIDS through IV drug use, transfusions, or sexual activity. By 1991, it is estimated that there will be 7,000 cases of AIDS transmitted by heterosexual contact (34).

Heterosexual transmission of AIDS occurs in Africa where it has been documented by many researchers. This fact should serve as a clear warning to sexually active individuals to limit their number of sexual contacts, use condoms or other barrier-type contraceptives to prevent transmission of the disease, and for married couples to remain monogamous.

Prostitutes, with or without a history of IV drug use, have been demonstrated to be transmitters of the AIDS virus in Africa (30). In the United States they also present a danger. In Miami, for example, 40 percent of 25 female prostitutes were reported to give positive tests for the AIDS antibodies in a CDC report dated December 6, 1985 (36), and similar results have also been reported from New York and Los Angeles. Male prostitutes servicing gay men would be at great risk to themselves as well as to their "Johns" unless preventative measures were always employed.

Five positive accomplishments in the battle with are demonstrating that the hepatitis B vaccine is not a transmission agent for AIDS, that the Factor VIII clotting agent needed for hemophilia treatment could be made safe by a heat treating process, identifying the HTLV-III virus as the causative agent for AIDS, the development of the ELISA test for detecting AIDS antibodies in blood, and progress made in determining the structure of the AIDS virus and its method of infection.

AIDS Assistance Organizations

If no one ever remarked, "Great crises beget great virtues," they ought to have, because over 1,000 organizations in the United States are now offering assistance, information, counseling, hospice care, legal services, social and life maintenance support to AIDS victims and their families. Almost every major city has an AIDS hotline to refer concerned individuals to appropriate information and services.

Programs administered by these groups have a diversity of approaches like the production of a 40-minute explicit film produced by the Gay Men's Health Crisis of New York to help popularize "safer sex." This film is designed to be used as one segment of a three-part educational program which also includes a question and answer session (Gay Men's Health Crisis, Inc., Box 272, New York, NY 10011).

AID Atlanta disseminates a newsletter, mans a hot line, offers discussion groups, and also incorporates "safer sex" demonstrations as part of their prevention program (AID Atlanta, 811 Cypress Street, N.E., Atlanta, GA 30308).

One of the earliest, and still one of the most successful, programs has been developed by the Shanti Project in San Francisco. This program incorporates a holistic approach in supporting the person who has AIDS, his friends and family by providing not only counseling and educational services but also providing emotional, social, legal, and living skills designed to help the person with AIDS maintain his independence as long, or as often, as he is able to do so (Shanti Project, 890 Hayes St., San Francisco, CA 94110).

PWA, the National Association of People With AIDS, has been formed as an advocate group to help protect the civil rights of those who have AIDS, to provide support to their members, and to help insure that those who have the syndrome have a voice in the design and administration of programs that may influence their lives. Perhaps the watchword of this organization is "empowerment." The meaning of this term was explained by a member of the organization with the statement, "We may be sick, but we are not helpless. We insist on controlling as much as we can of our lives. What we can do for ourselves, we want to do for ourselves. We feel it is our right to be informed of the details of any treatment, and the progress, or lack of progress, of any therapy. In sum, we insist on having input on decisions that affect our lives." (National Association of People With AIDS, P.O. Box 65472, Washington, D.C. 20035).

The National AIDS Network serves as a central organization for the exchange of information and materials as well as monitoring national and state legislation. This network is funded by the contributions from member AIDS-activity groups throughout the nation (National AIDS Network, 729 8th Street, S.E., Washington D.C. 20003).

The Lambda Legal Defense Fund monitors legislation as well as participates in court cases where the civil rights of those with AIDS have been abused (132 West 43rd Street, New York, New York 10036).

The majority of these organizations are manned by a largely volunteer staff. They may be sponsored by state or city public health departments, gay-lesbian action groups, charitable organizations, religious groups, or nonaffiliated private funding. Many of the staffs of volunteer organizations are gay, and some are ARC or AIDS patients themselves who can speak from personal experience about the disease. Others have had friends or lovers who have succumbed to AIDS and find volunteer work a useful catharsis in helping to overcome their loss.

One of the earliest groups to become active in providing support services for those with AIDS were members of already-organized lesbian groups whose members are among the least likely to contract AIDS because of their sexual practices. "This was done to help our brothers," remarked Caitlin Ryan, president of the National Lesbian and Gay Health Foundation (37). Such selfless dedication is common to many participants in AIDS organizations.

Other groups are now becoming active in AIDS education and prevention. Included among these is the American Red Cross which in 1986 was starting their AIDS program.

Still, some segments of the population in the United States are underserved. Among the groups that have not been reached as successfully as might be desired are Hispanic Americans, Black Americans, IV drug users, women, and the young.

Because of cultural differences, some Hispanic and Black Americans are reluctant to approach the nearly all-white, middle class AIDS organizations for assistance. Although appeals have been made to bring more minority groups into AIDS-assistance organizations, these segments of the population have not been adequately reached. In addition, there is a delay in producing up-to-date Spanish-language materials for American use, although efforts are being made by several organizations to correct this deficiency.

IV drug users are not organized, and reaching this segment of the population is difficult except through the segment of this group that uses methadone-maintenance clinics. In some states, and in the Netherlands, there is an exchange program where used needles and syringes may be swapped with no questions asked. Such programs reduce the spread of AIDS from contaminated injection equipment, provide a place where information can be distributed, and assist those wishing to "kick the habit." On a world-wide basis, the needle exchange program has been the most successful approach for reducing the spread of AIDS among IV drug users.

Sexually active individuals, of all ages, need information about AIDS prevention. Since many of the young began sexual experimentation during their teens, educational materials on AIDS need to be designed for this segment of the population. A publicly-funded school in the United States can usually offer information about the biological aspects of sex and prevention of diseases, but

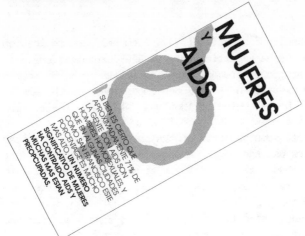

Figure 7. Women and AIDS, a Spanish-language flyer dis-
    tributed by the San Francisco Women's AIDS Network.
    This publication and others like them are needed to
    provide AIDS information to Hispanics, women and
    minority populations in the United States.

cannot comment on the spiritual or emotional aspects of
sex, as these issues touch on morality and/or religious
teachings. Popular magazines emphases the performance or
pleasurable aspects of sex but mostly ignore moral issues.

It is not surprising that spiritual/moral aspects of
sex have been largely overlooked, particularly in regards
to homosexuality and AIDS. In the case of a homosexual
with AIDS who is facing death, it is not unexpected that
he would seek spiritual comfort, despite the hostility of
main-stream religions towards homosexuality.

In seeking to reconcile himself he may abandon organized religion and seek his own way into spirituality
or embrace various aspects of Eastern religions.   Or, he
may try to reestablish connections with his previous
faith.   Whatever path a person might chose to follow to
spirituality must be first, his own choice and, secondly,
regarded with tolerance by those around him.

This private search into the meanings of life and
death is not one that can easily be presented as a universal "AIDS Action Program for Spiritual Development,"

but counselors should be aware, and not impede, any person's search for spiritual comfort.

Jim D'Eramo, former medical editor and science writer for "The New York Native," spoke at the Second International Conference on AIDS. He described a situation where a person with AIDS informed a professional psychosocial counselor that he had discovered God and how that revelation helped him in coping with AIDS. The counselor, gave the young man no encouragement, D'Eramo said, because religion had no place in the program she had outlined for her support group (38).

D'Eramo commented, "What arrogance she had to think that what she could offer was better than God....In my own experience those who have gone through the experience spiritually seem to be less impeded, less demoralized, and more at peace (than those who have not)."

The World Federation of Hemophilia with its offices in Heidelberg (c/o Stiftung Rehabilitation, Postfach 101409, 6900 Heidelberg 1, Federal Republic of Germany) serves as a compiler and disseminator of information about hemophilia. This organization has assembled and is constantly updating a 200-plus-page annotated bibliography on AIDS that is available to researchers.

Naively assuming that there were perhaps a hundred AIDS-support organizations when the first edition of this book was in preparation, it was thought that a listing might be included; but such a listing is a book-length work itself and is available from the National Lesbian and Gay Health Foundation, Inc. (NLGHF) at P.O. Box 65472, Washington, D.C. 20035 at a cost of $10.00.

One of the best documents on AIDS has been issued by the Orange County Health Care Agency and the University of California Irvine Medical Center. This publication, <u>Living With AIDS</u>, is available from the Gay & Lesbian Community Services Center, 12832 Garden Grove Boulevard, Suite E., Garden Grove, California 92643, for $12.00. Although some information in the book is now outdated (A problem with all AIDS publications, including this book.), it remains an excellent work that is well suited for use as a model for developing community health guides.

Another book, <u>Living With AIDS</u>: <u>A Self-Care Manual</u>, outlines practical approaches to enable a person with AIDS to cope with the syndrome. It may be ordered from AIDS Project Los Angeles, Inc., 7362 Santa Monica Boulevard, West Hollywood, California 90046 for $5.75 plus 6 percent state tax for in-state orders.

A collection of 25 papers presented at the first International Conference on AIDS is available from the Business Office, Annals of Internal Medicine, 4200 Pine Street, Philadelphia, Pennsylvania 19104, for $7.00.

Announcements have been made for the third and fourth international conferences on AIDS. The third conference is scheduled for Washington, D.C., for June of 1987, and the fourth will be held in Oslo, Sweden, in 1988. Information about the 1987 conference may be obtained from the International Conference on AIDS, 655 15th Street, N.W., Washington D.C. 20005, U.S.A.

---

1. Shilts, Randy, 1984, 70,000 gay men in San Francisco, first big study says: The San Francisco Chronicle, November 15.
2. Anonymous personal communication.
3. Montagnier, Luc, 1985, Lymphadenopathy/AIDS virus; from molecular structure to pathogenicity: Viral Oncology Unit, Pasteur Institute, Paris, France; International Conference on AIDS, Atlanta, Georgia.
4. Centers for Disease Control, 1982, Update on Kaposi's sarcoma and opportunistic infections in previously healthy persons -- United States: Centers for Disease Control, Atlanta, Georgia, June 11.
5. Centers for Disease Control, 1981, <u>Pneumocystis</u> pneumonia - Los Angeles: Morbidity and Mortality Weekly Report, Centers for Disease Control, Atlanta, Georgia, June 5.
6. Centers for Disease Control, 1981, Update on acquired immune deficiency syndrome (AIDS) - United

States: Morbidity and Mortality Weekly Report,
Centers for Disease Control, Atlanta, Georgia,
September 24.

7. Jaffe, Harold W., 1985, The epidemiology of AIDS in
homosexual men: Centers for Disease Control,
Atlanta, Georgia, International Conference on
AIDS, Atlanta, Georgia.

8. McCarthy, Kathy, 1985, Taking us off AIDS list can't
lift stigma: The Miami Herald, April 11.

9. Centers for Disease Control, 1982, Acquired immune
deficiency syndrome (AIDS); precautions for
clinical and laboratory staffs: Mortality Weekly Report, Centers for Disease Control, Atlanta, Georgia, November 5.

10. Centers for Disease Control, 1982, Possible Transfusion-associated acquired immune deficiency syndrome (AIDS) - California: Mortality Weekly
Report, Centers for Disease Control, Atlanta,
Georgia, December 10.

11. Centers for Disease Control, 1983, Immunodeficiency
among female sexual partners of males with
acquired immune deficiency syndrome (AIDS) --
New York: Mortality Weekly Report, Centers for
Disease Control, Atlanta, Georgia, January 7.

12. Centers for Disease Control, 1983, Prevention of acquired immune deficiency syndrome (AIDS);
Report of Inter-Agency Recommendations: Mortality Weekly Report, Centers for Disease Control,
Atlanta Georgia, March 4.

13. Centers for Disease Control, 1983, Acquired immuno-
deficiency syndrome (AIDS) -- Europe: Mortality
Weekly Report, Centers for Disease Control,
Atlanta, Georgia, September 9.

14. Shilts, Randy, 1984, The Intercontinental laboratory
war: San Francisco Chronicle, December 9.

15. Gallo, Robert C., 1985, The molecular biology and
antigenic structure of HTLV-III: National Cancer Institute, National Institutes of Health,
Bethesda, Maryland, International Conference on
AIDS, Atlanta, Georgia.

16. Centers for Disease Control, 1984, Update; acquired immunodeficiency syndrome (AIDS) - Europe: Mortality Weekly Report, Centers for Disease Control, Atlanta, Georgia, November 2.

17. Brunet, Jean-Baptiste, 1985, The international occurrence of AIDS: World Health Organization Collaborating Center for AIDS, Paris, France, International Conference on AIDS, Atlanta, Georgia.

18. Centers for Disease Control, 1985, Update; acquired immunodeficiency syndrome -- Europe: Mortality Weekly Report, Centers for Disease Control, Atlanta, Georgia, January 18.

19. Curran, James W., 1985, The epidemiology and prevention of AIDS: Center for Infectious Diseases, Centers for Disease Control, International Conference on AIDS, Atlanta, Georgia.

20. Seabrook, Charles, 1985, The deadly race against time; two million exposed, but no cure in sight: The Atlanta Journal-Constitution, September 8.

21. Centers for Disease Control, 1985, Update; acquired immunodeficiency syndrome -- United States: Mortality Weekly Report, Centers for Disease Control, Atlanta, Georgia, August 1.

22. Mahler, H., 1986, World Health Organization's programme on AIDS: World Health Organization, Second International Conference on AIDS, Paris, France.

23. Escoffier-Lambiotte, 1986, En Europe, le nombre de cas a augmente de 163 % en un an: Le Monde, Paris, France, June 25.

24. Wangroongsarb, Y., 1986, Prevalence of HTLV-III/LAV antibody in selected populations in Thailand: Second International Conference on AIDS, Paris, France.

25. Yeoh, E.K., 1986, Epidemiology of LAV-HTLV III infection in Hong Kong: Medical and Health Dept., Hong Kong; Second International Conference on AIDS, Paris, France.

26. Anonymous, 1986, AIDS reported from U.S.S.R.: Associated Press, June 27.

27. Brunet, J.B., 1986, AIDS in 1986; a worldwide health challenge: Second International Conference on AIDS, Paris, France.

28. Kapita, B.M., 1986, AIDS in Africa: Mama Yemo Hospital, Kinshasa, Zaire, Second International Conference on AIDS, Paris, France.

29. Mann, Johathan, M, 1986, Sexual practices associated with LAV/HTLV-III seropositivity among female prostitutes in Kinshasa, Zaire: Centers for Disease Control, Atlanta, Georgia, Second International Conference on AIDS, Paris, France.

30. Piot, P., 1986, Transmission patterns of LAV/HTLV III: evidence for heterosexual transmission: Institute of Tropical Medicine, Antwerp, Belgium; Project SIDA, Dinshasa, Zaire; Centers for Disease Control, Atlanta, Georgia; Second International Conference on AIDS, Paris, France.

31. Desmyter, J., 1986, Anti-LAV/HTLV-III in Kinshasa mothers in 1970 and 1980: Rega Institute, University of Leuven, Leuven, Belgium and Pasteur Institute, Paris, France; Second International Conference on AIDS, Paris, France.

32. Clavel, F., 1986, A new retrovirus in West African AIDS patients: Institut Pasteur, Paris, France; Hopital Claude Bernard, Paris, France; Ministere de la Sante, Lisbonne, Portugal; Second International Conference on AIDS, Paris, France.

33. Alizon, Marc, 1986, Molecular analysis of two AIDS virus isolates from Zairian patients: Unite d'Oncologie Virale, Institut Pasteur, Paris, France, Second International Conference on AIDS, Paris, France.

34. Curran, J.W., 1986, The epidemiology of AIDS; current status and future prospects: Centers for Disease Control, Second International Conference on AIDS, Paris, France.

35. Centers for Disease Control, 1986, Update, acquired, immunodeficiency syndrome - United States: Weekly Mortality Report, Centers for Disease Control, Atlanta, Georgia, January 13.

36. Centers for Disease Control, 1985, Recommendations for assisting in the prevention of perinatal transmission of human T-lymphotropic virus type III/lymphadenopathy-associated virus and acquired immunodeficiency syndrome: Weekly Mortality Report, Centers for Disease Control, Atlanta, Georgia, December 6.

37. Ryan, Caitlin, C, 1986, Opening address: Seventh National Lesbian/Gay Health Conference & Fourth National AIDS Forum, Washington, D.C., March 13.

38. Van Wijngaarden, Jan, K., 1986, AIDS policy co-ordination in the Netherlands: Polderweg 92, 1093 K p , Amsterdam, the Netherlands.

39. D'Eramo, Je, 1986, "800 Men"--a research, education and demonstration program for AIDS prevention in New York City: Second International Conference on AIDS, Paris, France.

THE AIDS VIRUS

THE STRUCTURE OF THE AIDS VIRUS is better known than it was a year ago. Although new discoveries continue to be made about retroviruses, and the AIDS virus in particular, the most important genetic components of the virus have been identified, the basic method of cell infectivity has been established, and work is under way to determine which gene determines what function of the virus.

From earlier work by Robert C. Gallo and others, all retroviruses are known to contain three virus genes necessary for reproduction, the Group Antigen (Gag), Polymerase (Pol), and Envelope (Env). The simplest known retrovirus which infects humans, HTLV-I (one of two known viruses which cause leukemia), contains these three genes. They are flanked on the left side of the genome (the 3' end) by a Long Terminal Repeat Sequence, LTR, and on the right side of the genome (the 5' end) by another Long Terminal Repeat sequence. HTLV-I also contains the Tat, Transactivating Transcription gene, which activates the expression of all the viral genes.

In HTLV-I and II, the Tat gene also activates expression of human cellular genes important to T-cell growth. This may be one method by which these retroviruses can cause leukemia in man (8).

HTLV-I

5'LTR / Gag / Pol /Envelope / Tat/ 3'LTR

In contrast to the relatively simple configuration of HTLV-I, HTLV-III/LAV (HIV) contains at least four additional genes. These are a Short Open Reading Frames (SOR) located between the Pol and the Tat gene, which includes a new gene named Tat III; an additional Short

Open Reading Frame after the Envelope gene on the 3' end
of the genome; and another Transacting gene, Trs, in the
same sequence as the Tat III gene (8).

The Gag, Pol, and Env genes of HTLV-III/LAV (HIV)
are similar to those of other human retroviruses, but the
Trs, Tat, Sor, and 3'Orf genes are structurally unique
(2). The Tat III gene has been found by M. Fisher to be
an absolute requirement for virus replacation as is the
Trs gene (1,8).   The Trs gene is in the same sequence as
the Tat III gene, but becaue it begans from a different
reading frame a different protein is made (8).

HTLV-III/LAV (HIV)

5'LTR/ Gag / Pol / Sor /Tat(Trs)/Envelope /3'Orf /3'LTR

Each of these genes is composed of one or more
proteins which are identified by their molecular weights.
The molecular weight of these proteins is important because of their ability or reluctance to move through a
gel under the response of an electrical current in tests
such as the Western Blot.   Proteins identified from the
various genes of the HTLV-III/LAV (HIV) virus genome are
listed in table 8.

This genomic sequence in the viral RNA contains all
the necessary information for the virus to reproduce once
it enters the host cell.   Determining the function of
each genetic component is necessary to an understanding
of how the virus works and how to defeat it.   Present
techniques in microbiology allow individual genes to be
isolated and reproduced so that the functions of individual genes can be examined.

Gene substitutions can be used to determine possible
approaches of blocking a vital gene with a drug and
killing the virus or substituting an inert gene into the
viral structure that will enable a harmless form of the
virus to reproduce.   An inert viral form could cause the
body to produce large numbers of protective antibodies,

Table 8.   Molecular weight of proteins identified with
           the HTLV III (HIV) virus genome.

Gene Name	Primary Proteins	Derivative proteins
Envelope gene	GP 160 (150)	GP 120 (110) GP 41
3' Orf	P 27 P 23	
Gag gene	P 55	P 24 P 17 P 15
Tat gene		
Sor gene		
Pol gene	P 6, P 56 (duplex) P 34	

and provide a basis for a vaccine or therapy for AIDS.

The Gag gene provides the genetic information for
making the proteins in the core of the virus, the Pol,
coding for the formation of the reverse transcriptase
enzyme   which is necessary for virus reproduction,
and the Env, the genetic coding for making the virus'
glycoprotein envelope.

The Tat genes activate the transcription of the
viral RNA to DNA once the virus has entered the host
cell.   Once activated, Gallo has found that the Tat gene
of the leukemia virus (HTLV-I) caused the body to produce
large amounts of interleukin 2 (the T-cell growth factor). With HTLV-III/LAV (HIV), immune stimulation of the
T-cell leads to Tat gene expression and eventually the
Trs gene. The protein products of these genes causes a
tremendous burst of replication which Gallo maintains is

the most important cause of T-cell death. He also discovered that the Env protein was primarily responsible for the formation of giant multinucleated cells. Gallo stated that although muntinucleated cell formation ultimately resulted in the death of T-4 cells, this method was not the most important cause of T-cell death or the explosive proliferation of the virus (3). The death of T-4 cells is the primary means that the T-4 to T-8 cell ratio in the blood becomes unbalanced.

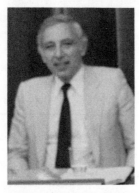

Gallo said that he suspected that other, yet undiscovered, viruses might be important in cancers, such as KS and lymphomas, seen in AIDS because the viral genes of HTLV-III/LAV (HIV) could not be detected in these cancers (3). Since the first isolation of LAV in France and HTLV-III in the United States, it was recognized that the virus exhibited a great deal of genetic variability. Gallo observed that the viruses differed by as much as 80 to 1,200 nucleotides from from sample to sample. This variation occurs not only in samples of the virus from different parts of the world, but also, to a lessor degree, in time in infected individuals. Gallo maintained that such a natural variability in the virus might explain why macrophages, particularly in the brain, are favored hosts for the HTLV III/LAV (HIV) virus whereas elsewhere in the body the T-4 cells are the preferred hosts (3).

Figure 8. Robert C. Gallo of the National Institutes of Health, Bethesda, Maryland.

OTHER HUMAN RETROVIRUSES

The discovery of HTLV IV and LAV 2 in 1986 opened new areas of retrovirus investigation. In describing

LAV 2, Luk Montagnier, reported that this virus had been isolated from West Africa, and had pathological effects similar to frank AIDS (4). The same author reported that the virus crossreacts weakly with his original isolate of LAV I (HIV) indicating that the two viruses have some genetic material in common. The LAV 2 virus has been detected in one French blood sample that was taken from a man who had a West African wife. Clavel, of the Pasteur Institute, reported that LAV 2 was not detected by the ELISA or Western Blot tests developed for the AIDS virus.

Gallo, referring to HTLV IV, said that the pathologic effects or viral genome of this virus had not been determined, but that during the next year these questions ought to be answered (3).

An antibody so similar to the AIDS antibody that it gives a positive Western Blot test result was found by F. Merino of the Venezuelan Institute of Scientific Investigation in that country's native populations. The antibodies were detected in blood samples from healthy and ill (malaria and Chagas' disease) Indians in Amazonia (6). None of about 170 random, healthy blood donors from seven Venezuelan cities were found to host the viral antibodies (6).

A similar antibody response has been achieved from testing of blood samples from three Cree Indian children from an isolated village in northern Canada. C. Tsoukas found that blood taken from three surviving children out of nine which exhibited AIDS-like symptoms had positive ELISA tests for the AIDS antibodies (7).

Gallo recommended caution in accepting these results at face value until these virus cultures from the Americas could be examined (8).

----

1. Fisher, Amanda G., 1965, The trans-activator gene of HTLV-III (TAT-III) is essential for HTLV-III replication; evidence from transfection studies using a biologically active molecular clone: Laboratory of Tumor Cell Biology, Developmental

Therapeutics Program, National Cancer Institute, National Institutes of Health, Bethesda, Maryland; Second International Conference on AIDS, Paris, France.

2. Ratner, Lee, 1986, Complete nucleotide sequence of functional clones of the virus associated with the acquired immunodeficiency syndrome, HTLV-III/LAV: Division of Hematology and Oncology, Washington University, St. Louis, Mo.; Laboratory of Tumor Cell Biology, National Cancer Institute, Bethesda, Md.; and Biotech Research Laboratories, Inc, Rockville, Md.; Second International Conference on AIDS, Paris, France.

3. Gallo, Robert C., 1986, Human retroviruses, now and the future: National Institutes of Health, Bethesda, Maryland; Second International Conference on AIDS, Paris, France.

4. Montagnier, Luc, 1986, The AIDS virus; an update: Viral Oncology Unit, Pasteur Institute, Paris, France; Second International Conference on AIDS, Paris, France.

5. Clavel, F., 1986, A new retrovirus in West African AIDS patients: Institut Pasteur, Paris, France; Second International Conference on AIDS, Paris, France.

6. Merino, F., 1986, Anti-HTLV-III/LAV antibodies among native populations in Venezuela: Dept. of Pathology & Microbiology, UNMC, Omaha, Nebraska; Dept. Experimental Medicine, Instituto Venezolano de Investigations Cientificas, Caracas, Venezuela; Second International Conference on AIDS, Paris, France.

7. Tsoukas, C., 1986, A possible retroviral related neurologic disease among isolated Cree Indians: Montreal General Hospital and Montreal Children's Hospital, Montreal, Canada; Second International Conference on AIDS, Paris, France.

8. Gallo, Robert C., 1986, Personal communication: National Institutes of Health, Bethesda, Maryland, Sept. 17.

TRANSMISSION OF AIDS

TRANSMISSION OF AIDS occurs on at least four levels
of activity: 1. from person to person, 2. from virus to
cell, 3. within the cell, and 4. from cell to cell. If
any of these transmission paths can be interrupted, the
disease, under ideal circumstances, would not spread beyond those who are already infected.

PERSON-TO-PERSON

Sexual transmission is the most common method of
spreading the AIDS virus. Although statistics vary somewhat from year to year, about 73 percent of AIDS-infected
individuals in the United States were exposed to the
virus through sexual activities. The second most common
mode of infection was needle use among IV drug users,
which presently averages about 17 percent of this country's AIDS cases. The percentage of AIDS-infected individuals exposed through blood transfusions or blood products is usually about 2 percent (1). A less common mode
of transmission is from infected mothers to their newborn
children.

One advance in AIDS prevention was the discovery
that the AIDS viruses in the Factor VIII blood extracts
used for preventing bleeding episodes in hemophiciacs
could be killed by heat treatment. All Factor VIII
produced in the United States is now safe, but this is
little comfort to the 162 hemophiliacs in this country
and the 53 in Europe who are presumed to have contracted
AIDS from the contaminated product (2, 30).

Another significant advance in prevention was the
development of the ELISA test for detecting AIDS antibodies in blood samples. All new blood taken in and all
blood in United States blood banks have been screened,
and over 1,484 units of AIDS-virus-bearing blood were

detected out of 593,831 units tested in April and May of 1985 (3). Gays, bisexuals, IV drug users, those with ARC or AIDS, and men who had a single homosexual sex encounter as early as eight years ago continue to be asked not to donate blood as an additional precaution (4). As a result, the risk to the recipient of a blood transfusion has been greatly reduced.

A select panel of the National Institutes of Health met at Bethesda, Maryland, in July of 1986 and made three recommendations concerning blood donations: 1. A donor could designate that his blood be used for research purposes only. 2. Those seeking an elective surgical procedure would be encouraged to stockpile their own blood for allogenous transfusions. 3. Blood banks should inform donors if their blood was found to give ambiguous results with ELISA testing (31). (Donors are notified in most states if their blood gives a positive test result for the AIDS virus.)

An adverse result of the news about AIDS-contaminated blood supply was that some of those who were not members of risk groups discontinued donating blood out of fear of catching AIDS (5). The Red Cross, United States Public Health Service, and the World Health Organization are unanimous in their opinions that there is no risk to the donor when he gives blood as sterile, disposable equipment is used.

Joint bleeding is one of the most severe and disabling problems confronting hemophiliacs. A therapy used to prevent bleeding is to periodically administer the clotting factor as a preventative measure. R. Madhok of the Glasgow Royal Infirmary, Scotland, stated at the Second International Conference on AIDS that hemophiliacs were waiting until bleeding episodes occurred before seeking treatment, despite the availability of AIDS-virus-free blood products since October, 1985 (32).

F.R. Rosendaal of the Dutch Hemophilia Society perhaps best stated this behavioral change when he remarked, "A fairly large number (of hemophiliac patients have) made changes in their therapy schedule of which the protective effect is to be questioned (33)."

Other centers treating hemophiliacs have witnessed a similar reluctance of their patients to prophylaxis treatment. In centers where heat-treated clotting factors are universally used, the slight, if any, risk is acceptable. In developing countries where blood products may be of doubtful origin or were produced before heat treatment of clotting factors was instituted, a degree of risk may remain.

Of concern to health care workers is their chances of being infected with AIDS by a patient. While it cannot be claimed that there is no risk, these risks are very small and can be reduced to nearly nil if proper precautions are taken. To date, no health care personnel who were not in risk groups have contracted AIDS, although two did test positive for the virus (one after a needle-stick injury and the other after a cut sustained while handling blood (6)).

In following 300 health care workers with repeated intense exposure to AIDS patients in the AIDS unit of San Francisco General Hospital, only one, a homosexual man with admitted risk factors, tested positively for the virus. This result was obtained despite a total of 315 accidental needlesticks or mucosal splashes with AIDS-contaminated blood or body fluids. This study, reported by J. Louise Gerberding, concluded that, "Health care workers are at minimal risk for acquiring AIDS virus from occupational exposure (34)."

Casual contact is an issue being hotly debated in the nation's courts. Can a child with AIDS be allowed to go to school where some fear he might infect other children (7)? This question will be heard in courts all over the country and is a concern that must be resolved on an individual basis. The proper answer will depend on the age of the child, his temperament, and what symptoms the child is exhibiting at the time (8).

An active mind can conjure up any number of possible, if unlikely, circumstances where an expert sitting on the witness stand during a court trial would have to say, "Yes, AIDS could possibly be transmitted like this, but ...."

"I'm sorry sir, but I believe you have answered my question," the examining attorney would interject before the witness could add the qualifier that this was an unlikely event.

A child with AIDS could transmit the disease to his fellow students in the same manner as do adults; i.e., fluid-sharing sex and using contaminated needles to take drugs.

"But what about a smaller child, could he bite another child and give him AIDS?"

In an August, 1985, release the CDC said that casual contact in schools was not likely to result in the transmission of AIDS, but stopped short of stating that such transmission could never occur (8). There is perhaps a slight risk to the close associates and playmates of an infected child, but none to those in other classes in the school who might occasionally pass him in the hall.

Several aspects of this problem were approached at the epidemiologic sessions of the Second International Conference on AIDS. Claude Griscelli of the Hospital of Infant Diseases in Paris estimated that there were about 200 children with AIDS in the United States and approximately 60 in Europe (35). In a study by Martha F. Rogers of the CDC, 35 family members, including ten children with transfusion-associated AIDS, who had lived together and shared many household items for an average of 21 months were tested. In this study no evidence of AIDS transmission was found between the children to other siblings or adult family members (36).

The issue of biting was addressed in a paper given by H. W. Jaffe who described an aggressive, deranged AIDS patient who during his course of treatment bit and/or scratched health care workers with bloody or feces-fouled fingers. Even in this intense-contact situation no transmission of the AIDS virus was observed (37).

The nature and levels of risk can perhaps be categorized something like the following table indicates. This table is offered merely to aid in the discussion of the orders of magnitude of risk for various activities.

Somewhere below the last category would be listed

Table 9. Supposed risk factors in sexual and health care activities.*

Risk	Verbal interpretation	Activity
1:1	A sure thing.	Repeated penetrative anal sex with a number of infected partners over a prolonged period.
1:2	Very high risk.	Repeated penetrative anal sex with one infected partner.
1:10	High risk.	Repeated penetrative anal sex with a number of anonymous partners.
1:50	At risk.	Needle sharing I.V. drug users.
1:100	Moderate risk.	Repeated penetrative anal sex with multiple partners, but using a condom.
1:1,000	Small risk.	Avoiding penetrative sex, but still engaging in semen-external body contact.
1:10,000	Slight risk	Avoiding penetrative sex, semen, saliva and body waste contact, but engaging in mutual masturbation.
1:1,000,000	Very slight risk.	Nurse in intensive care ward exclusively treating AIDS patients who mostly follows safe-care guidelines, but may have rare, external exposure to body fluids.
1:10,000,000	Almost no risk.	Nurse in intensive care ward exclusively treating AIDS patients who always follows safe-care guidelines.

* Expressed as approximate orders of magnitude.

casual contact between individuals, the risk to hospital workers in other wards of the hospital and the risk to the general public; but these risk factors are hypothetical. Detailed, scientifically supportable risk analysis awaits thousands of case studies before dependable numbers can be assigned.

Sexual Transmission

This category of transmission is where the most danger lies for the uninfected individual and where education and behavioral modifications can reduce the rate of spread of AIDS. Changes in sex habits could only be expected to decrease the number of AIDS cases that would develop in two-to-five years and not immediately halt the yearly doubling of the number of AIDS cases in the U.S. (9). Individuals now progressing to AIDS were those who were mostly infected before "Safer Sex" guidelines had been developed.

Because no obvious, immediate benefits to the individuals who have modified their sex habits will be seen, it will be difficult to sustain a prevention program over the number of years it will take before the first reduction in the rate of spread of AIDS is seen (10). Anything becomes stale through repetition, and fresh approaches will be necessary to sustain the effectiveness of prevention programs. It will also be increasingly difficult to persuade local governments to continue financing AIDS prevention programs when indications of positive results are so long delayed.

Despite increasing amounts of federal fundings for AIDS research, budgets for AIDS organizations at the the local level are largely unable to cope with the demand for services, information, and social support.

The development of "Safer Sex" guidelines fell by default to state and local public health departments and gay organizations because of an apparent reluctance of the United States Department of Health and Human Services to investigate preventative measures to slow the

the sexual transmission of AIDS. At the First International Conference on AIDS, criticism was directed against Margaret Heckler, former Secretary of the Department of Health and Human Services, by gay service groups for her department's not moving more aggressively into the investigation of methods of having safer sex and documenting the safety of condoms in preventing the spread of AIDS.

Perhaps out of a fear of appearing to promote gay sex at a time when a conservative administration was sitting in the White House, the department at the time of the First International Conference was distributing only one 16-page piece of cartoon-illustrated literature, "What Gay and Bisexual Men Should Know about AIDS,"

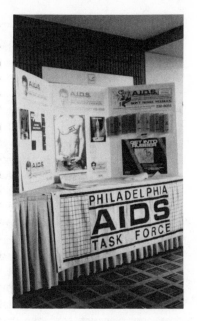

Figure 9. Philadelphia AIDS Task Force exhibit at the First International Conference on AIDS. Among the literature offered were pocket cards, a display urging condom use and a warning to not share needles.

directed at preventing the sexual spread of AIDS among these risk groups, compared to a variety of cards, ads, posters, billboards, booklets, and books numbering in the hundreds exhibited by others at the conference (11).

A step in promoting safer sexual activity was the CDC release of January 11, 1985, which stated that those with positive ELISA blood test for the AIDS virus should be informed that, "There is a risk of infecting others by sexual intercourse, sharing of needles, and possibly exposure of others to saliva through oral-genital contact or intimate kissing. The efficacy of condoms in preventing infection with HTLV-III is unproven, but the consistent use of them may reduce transmission (13)."

Marcus A. Conant of the University of California at San Francisco did a series of tests on three latex, one natural lambskin, and one synthetic skin condom. He confirmed that there was no transmission of virus through the condom materials (38). In addition, Bruce Voeller of the Mariposa Education and Research Foundation of Los Angeles found that weak concentrations of the spermicide nonoxynol-9 would kill the AIDS virus in cultures within 60 seconds. Voeller stated that this spermicide had been used safely in stronger concentrations in commercially available preparation for decades, and suggested that use of both a spermicide and condom would offer a higher degree of protection to both sex partners (39).

What effects the long term use of nonoxynol-9 might have during anal sex is not presently known. Voeller's comments on the safety of this product in vaginal sex does not assure that the product is also safe for anal sex. Gays have used this product anally, but its anal use could conceivably result in higher numbers of rectal cancers, or other problems, that might take years to develop. Additional study is needed to clear this product for anal use.

Condom use in vaginal sex is usually stated to be about 97 percent effective in preventing pregnancies. While a three percent failure rate is acceptable in birth control, it is not when the condom is the only block to a life-threatening disease.

Condom failure rates could be expected to be higher in anal sex because of added stress placed on the relatively thin membrane. In recognition of this, some makers are now offering condoms made of thicker materials. Because of wide variations in the size and shape of the erect penis (less than an inch long to in excess of 14 inches), the one-size-fits-all approach to condoms leaves those on both ends of the size scale with less than effective protection.

Different approaches have been taken for disseminating "Safer Sex" information to gays. A pocket card prepared by the San Francisco AIDS Foundation puts various sexual activities into three categories: Safe Sex, Possibly Safe Sex Practices, and Unsafe Sex Practices.

Safe Sex Practices: Massage, Hugging, Mutual Masturbation, Social Kissing (Dry), Body-to-Body Rubbing .

Possibly Safe Sex Practices: French Kissing (Wet), Anal Intercourse With Condom, Sucking - Stop Before Climax, Watersports - External Only.

Unsafe Sex Practices: Rimming, Fisting, Blood Contact, Sharing Sex Toys, Semen or Urine in Mouth, Anal Intercourse Without Condom.

The same information and a bit more is contained in an informational handout distributed by the AIDS Action Project of the Chicago Howard Brown Memorial Clinic (14). When discussing specific sexual activities, they made the following recommendations:

Hugging, cuddling, sexual massage. These activities are wonderfully sexual and do not involve the direct exchange of bodily fluids.

Kissing. If neither partner has open cuts or sores of the mouth, lips, or tongue, kissing probably presents little risk.

Mutual masturbation. Again, since no bodily fluids are exchanged, mutual masturbation probably offers no risk for AIDS transmission. However, be careful where you aim. Avoid eyes, mouth.

Use your imagination. Fantasy, visual sex (erotic movies).

The Brown Clinic guidelines also state, "Oral-genital sex and rectal intercourse may present somewhat greater risk for AIDS transmission, especially if semen is injected into the mouth or rectum. To possibly reduce your risk, pull out before you ejaculate.

"'Fisting' may be a high-risk activity. This is because it can produce small tears in the skin that lines the anus. These tears can allow infectious agents to qain direct access to your bloodstream or directly expose you to your partner's blood."

Insertion of the fist or contaminated sex toys

through the anus into the rectal cavity may be the single most risky sexual activity for the passive partner. This risk is greatly increased if fisting is preceded or followed by penis insertion with ejaculation. These circumstances would allow easy access to the bloodstream of both partners for any sexually transmitted infectious agents, including the AIDS virus, syphilis, or hepatitis. About the same risk would probably result from oral-anal contact preceding or following fisting or penis penetration with ejaculation.

The determination of the relative amount of risk from a one-time sexual encounter with an infected individual has not been made. Because of the long latent period between infection and the presentation of symptoms, this information may be unobtainable. Sex with the exchange of body fluids with a person who is, or may be, infected with AIDS should always be considered a high-risk activity.

There are people who have had sex with individuals and found out years later that their sex partner had developed AIDS. Many who have been potentially exposed to the AIDS virus do not give a positive test for the virus (15). This results indicate that either the virus is in the body and not undergoing much reproduction, hence too few antibodies are found in the blood to detect; that the individual already has an immune-suppression disease and no antibodies to the virus are being produced, although the virus is proliferating; that somehow the virus is encapsulated and not reproducing; that the virus was defeated by the body without producing antibodies; that the virus was not successfully transmitted; or that the sex partner had not been exposed at the time of the sexual contact.

Much less attention has been given to the prevention of virus transfer between heterosexual individuals than between male homosexuals (16). The use of condoms, spermacides, and the avoidance of oral-genital or oral-anal contact (either active or passive) would appear to be the best means of avoiding infection. Male-female, female-male or mutual masturbation would appear by anal-

ogy to existing guidelines for homosexuals to offer   less
risk provided that body fluids are not transmitted by the
hand to the mouth or eyes and the skin on the   hands   is
unbroken.

Safer Sex

Homosexuals

It is very difficult for people who test positively
for the AIDS virus, but have not expressed any symptoms
to accept that they must no longer have sex.   Likely,
many will not accept such a burden, and attempts to
demand that they cease sexual activity may result in
their engaging in more high risk sex, rather than less.

The only sure way to avoid sexually-transmitted
diseases is not to have sex, and a minority of seropositive individuals have chosen this option.   More have
resolved to reduce the number of sexual contacts, but
this is not an effective approach because of the increasing prevalence of AIDS-virus-infection   throughout the
world (40).

Avoiding not all sexual activity but all DANGEROUS
sexual activity is the most viable alternative to most
gays and heterosexuals who have been infected with the
virus and for those who wish to avoid being infected.   In
simple words, this means no fluid-exchange sex.

Gay Men's Health Crisis of New York has prepared an
explicit, erotic film showing gay safe-sex techniques
that they use as a segment of a three-part program on
AIDS.   The film is done to high professional standards
and ends with a poignant scene where a person with AIDS
and his lover confront the possibility of being parted.
This last scene is designed to bring the viewer down from
an erotic high and prepare him for a frank discussion of
the problems of AIDS which follows the film.

In New York and other cities there are "jack off"
(JO) parties where the participants stimulate each other,
but do not engage in penetrative sex or fluid exchange.

Heterosexuals

The above approaches work well with gays, but many heterosexuals would find these approaches, or pictorial representations of them, repugnant. Even the more broad-minded among them would probably reply, "These are fine for gays, but fellow, I ain't gay."

The "healthy sex" approaches can be adapted for use in a heterosexual context. Even if the spiritual and emotional aspects of sex are disregarded and only the sex act is considered, options like massage, playful bondage, masturbation, or just a good strong hug can do much towards establishing intimacy without penetrative sex.

Where penetrative sex is desired, condom use with spermicides can remove much of the risk for both partners. In addition, penetrative sex should be avoided after any type of genital infection or trauma, such as following childbirth, because under such conditions large numbers of T-4 cells would be expected to be present in the vaginal cavity or discharged with the ejaculate, which would increase the risk of infection.

The AIDS virus has been identified in the vaginal and cervical secretion of infected women, and Constance B. Wofsy of the University of California advised that "safe sex and condoms (be used by)...men and women at high risk (41). The avoidance of anal sex does not appear to result in an appreciable decrease in the chances of being infected by the virus based on present studies among African prostitutes (41).

A question of interest is how does one handle the situation when an attractive potential sexual partner is met and the decision is made to spend the night together? Does one pull out a printed form for the other to sign certifying that they are free of 17 venereal diseases and loose a lovely evening?

A better approach would be to keep some condoms and spermicide handy, and use them, with nothing said about it. Both partners would probably find this a more satisfactory approach in this era of rising incidences of sexually-transmitted diseases.

Another situation is that two people who have led active sex lives decide to marry, or began a long-term relationship. To acquire a marriage license, a blood test for syphilis is required. Might not the blood also be tested for AIDS? Some states may permit such tests if requested by both parties, but in none will it be automatically done. There are, however, anonymous testing sites where their privacy will be respected.

Protecting AIDS-antibody test results against unauthorized release is a legal problem that is receiving world-wide attention, but the basic premise has been generally accepted in the United States and Europe that these results are strictly confidential. Most states in the United States release results can be only to the person being tested or to his physician.

IV Drug Use

If ten percent of the nation's alcoholic beverages were contaminated with a poison that was known to lead to death within six months, there would still be those who would disregard the death threat and drink. Some would be alcoholics, but others would drink to... prove their manhood?...prove that they are still alive?...just be happy?...be one of the gang?...forget their troubles?

A similar situation exists with IV drug users. There are addicts and a larger population of occasional users (17). All of them should know from frequent examples that these drugs have a high potential for addiction and that heavy users of IV drugs have a reduced lifespan (18). To the addict, the danger of also contracting AIDS is part of the risk of sustaining an already deadly habit. The most promising group for risk reduction appears to be the occasional user (18).

To a person who does not use drugs, the idea of sharing a needle to inject himself and then inject others deserves a word of explanation. Often, the user is not a solitary person who uses some dark corner to inject himself. Several people will pool their money to make a buy. Then they will all go somewhere, make up the drug, and use a single needle and syringe to "fix" everyone who put money into the purchase. In this manner, a single needle may be used to rapidly inject a group of acquaintances. In a "shooting gallery," the chance of a patron being given a sterile needle and syringe is probably not very high, despite claims to the contrary.

The AIDS virus can apparently live so long as the medium (blood, urine, semen, etc.) is wet. When it is exposed to air, the virus may survive for several hours, but ultimately dies. As long as blood remains in or on the needle, that needle must be considered capable of transmitting the virus. If a person is going to inject himself with a drug, he should take pains to insure that he is using sterilized instruments and not share them.

This brings up the point of where does an addict obtain sterilized needles - not very often from the corner drugstore because he would expose himself as a user. In addition, arrests can be made for the possession of "drug paraphernalia" even if no drugs are found.

The result is that the user may know that he needs to use sterile equipment, but has no way to acquire the items without stealing them from a hospital, or risk possible arrest by buying them from a pharmacy, or purchasing needles of doubtful sterility from a street dealer or in a "shooting gallery." Should clinics treating drug abuse and sexually transmitted diseases dispense injection kits to users to attempt to reduce this route of AIDS transmission?

Some maintain that such an approach would be abetting rather than solving the problem of reducing the spread of AIDS among IV drug users. However, enforcement of present drug laws in the United States has not been noticeably effective in reducing the availability of street drugs. Although heroin lagged in popularity a bit as it was replaced by the more "socially acceptable" cocaine, its street use is now increasing as heroin is being promoted as a way to reduce the severity of the "crash" caused by crack, a highly addictive form of cocaine which is smoked. Both heroin and cocaine, alone or in combination with other drugs, are often injected.

Dutch authorities have begun a needle exchange program to help combat the spread of AIDS among drug users. Drug use in the Netherlands is illegal, but the Dutch have not ignored the problem. Among the materials exhibited at the Second International Conference on AIDS were handouts in English, French, and German prepared by the Amsterdam Municipal Public Health Service. These pamphlets warn of the dangers of drug use, the dangers of AIDS, and gives an easily remembered emergency number, seven 5s, to call if help is needed.

The needle-syringe exchange system was begun in Amsterdam in 1984 with two basic aims. The first was to prevent the spread of AIDS by providing sterile injection equipment with no questions asked, and the second, provide locations for promoting rehabilitation efforts (42).

Educational programs advising of the dangers of drug use need to be initiated at an early age to reduce the demand for drugs (18). Such programs will never be startlingly effective, given that the human animal is what he is, but at least the person offered drugs for the first time would know what he was getting into.

Organs, Blood, Blood Products and Body Waste

If a person has AIDS, ARC, or is infected with the virus and not exhibiting symptoms, his semen, blood, tears, saliva, organs, bone marrow, muscle tissues, urine, and stool may contain the virus and/or transmissible agents from opportunistic infections (8). To this list might also be added mother's milk (8) as well as any other body secretion, since all contain lymphocytes.

The amount of AIDS virus received, the quantity of inoculum, is seen as a possible determining factor in AIDS infection. Virus has been recovered from saliva, tears, and sweat; but in only small quantities. These fluids are not important transmitters of AIDS, but that is not the same as saying that they never transmit the virus (37). Insufficient evidence has been gathered to say that exposure to these fluids can never result in an AIDS infection, but those who fear that they may have contracted the virus with no contact other than kissing can sleep a great deal easier.

Evidence of transmission from stool and urine is not as clear. It would appear logical that bloody body waste present a greater danger than if no blood was being discharged, but this issue has received insufficient investigation. For safety's sake, these waste products should still be regarded as potentially infectious.

No person infected with the virus should be a blood, organ, or sperm donor (or in the case of a woman, a surrogate mother) for fear of transmitting the disease to others (4). Blood and semen contain high concentrations of the virus and are universally recognized as being the most important agents in transmitting AIDS. The virus has also been detected in women's vaginal-cervical secretions and these secretions probably serve as a media for AIDS transmission (41).

Organ transplants have become important in modern medical treatment. Organs must be removed from the donor and shipped very rapidly. Some organs are donated by healthy individuals, but most are from donors who are clinically dead. If the latter is the case, testing for the AIDS virus should be customarily done.

If a person is clinically dead, the possible disclosure of his AIDS antibody status would seem to be of little importance. If an otherwise willing donor should refuse, for any reason, to have his blood tested for the AIDS virus, there would be a risk of AIDS infection. This is particularly dangerous since the recipient often has his immune system chemically suppressed so that the new organ will not be rejected. Under such conditions, any virus contained in the organ would have a head start in an already weakened individual.

Any person whose job requires contact with any of the body products mentioned above, particularly when any blood might also be contained in them, should take reasonable precautions to protect himself (8).

VIRUS-TO-CELL

How the AIDS virus infects the cell has been an object of intense investigation since the identification of the HTLV-III/LAV (now designated HIV) virus as the causative agent of AIDS. Some of the mechanisms and their effects are still conjectural, but a much clearer understanding of the mechanisms of infection was presented by several authors at the Second International Conference on AIDS.

Free virus as well as a population of infected T-4 cells enters the body when it is inoculated with either blood or semen. Of the two, R.C. Gallo believes that the free virus is more important in generating infection in other cells, while W.A. Haseltine of Harvard Medical School is of the opinion that infected T-4 cells are the more important agent (43, 44).

Once in the bloodstream, the virus particles are scavenged by cells of the macrophage lineage. Virus reproduction may occur in macrophage, or macrophage-like cells, with or without causing disease. The carrier macrophages transport the virus to the lymph nodes where the macrophage cells are brought into contact with the follicular dendritic cells in the lymph nodes. There, the virus (as free virus?) comes in contact with the T-4 cells and infects them (43).

Some macrophages, particularly macrophage-like cells in the brain, are apparently continuously infected by the AIDS virus as virus may be isolated from these cells during all stages of infection; and the virus seemingly can also reproduce in these cells as well as in T-4 cells.

All T-4 cells contain in their genetic package retroviral genes and parts of retroviral genes. This genetic information is preserved each time the cell reproduces, but this contained genetic material does not cause disease. It is like fragments of a an incomplete blueprint to which additional pages must be added in order to form a complete plan for virus reproduction. These segments and bits of retroviral genes indicate that retrovirus infections in man, and primates, have been present for many human generations (45).

Viruses cannot reproduce by themselves. They must pirate genetic information from a host cell. By observation, it appears that both the T-4 and at least certain macrophage cells contain the needed elements that allow for AIDS virus reproduction. The virus, in order to reproduce, must inject its genetic information into an appropriate host cell, and this cell must have an appropriate receptor site to allow the crystalline virus to attach itself and penetrate the cell wall without killing the host cell.

WITHIN THE CELL

Within the cell, retroviral genes in the host cell are added to the injected genetic blueprint from the virus. When triggered by a poorly known factor/s, the enzyme reverse transcriptase is released, which causes the viral RNA to split and form the double-stranded DNA that the virus must have to reproduce. New viruses are budded from the infected cell. On occasion the new viruses explosively break through the cell wall, and the host cell dies. If reverse transcriptase activity is not present, the genetic information injected into the virus is preserved in the genome of the host cell and is reproduced with each cell division.

Some host T-4 cells become cancerous and form giant multinucleated cells in which virus reproduction also occurs. Gallo and Haseltine also differ whether this mechanism is the most important cause of deaths, and subsequent reductions in the numbers, of T-4 cells. Gallo admits that this process occurs, but believes that most of the mortality of T-cells is caused by their infection with the virus rather than due to giant cell formation (43).

Giant multinucleated cells have been found in virtually every organ of the body in advanced cases of AIDS with the virus count of some organs measuring in the millions of viruses per gram of tissue (27).

A key, unresolved question is what triggers the rapid reproduction of the virus seen in AIDS and why the virus often remains latent for years before rapid reproduction begins.

If Haseltine's model is accepted, cancerous giant cells are required to releases large quantities of the virus and infect other cells (44). If Gallo's model is correct, a cofactor, such as infection with another virus or other presently unrecognized agents, may weaken the T-4 cells and permit rapid virus reproduction in activated T-4 cells (43).

In the laboratory the AIDS virus cannot reproduce in healthy T-4 cells, but will only multiply in leukemic T-4 cells. If there is an analogy between laboratory results and that seen in man, it may be that a challenge to the T-4 cells by another agent, perhaps one of the opportunistic infections and perhaps not, is necessary to induce large-scale reproduction of the AIDS virus and deaths of large numbers of T-cells.

VIRUS KILLING AND VACCINE

If the AIDS viruses cannot be killed before they enter the body or in the bloodstream, preventing the virus from entering the T-4 cell would be the next possible step for the elimination of the AIDS virus (19).

If the virus cannot enter the cell, it cannot reproduce; and the few viruses in the bloodstream would be quickly destroyed. Two possible preventive approaches would be a drug to kill the virus in the bloodstream or to chemically block the "lock-on" sites on the virus that allows it to attach to the host cells. If the specific "lock on" sites on the virus can be filled with a non-toxic organic compound, the virus would be rendered sexually inert and unable to reproduce since it needs the genetic material inside the T-4 lymphocytes to multiply (20). Once bonded with the compound, the virus could be eliminated from the bloodstream as a waste product.

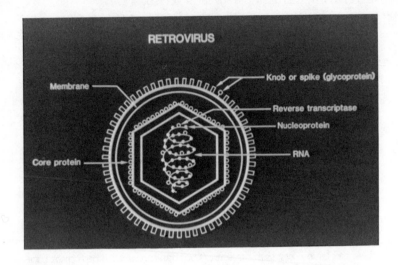

Figure 10. An idealized retrovirus showing glycoprotein
    envelope, RNA, and site of reverse transcriptase on
    RNA strand. Once genetic material has been pirated
    from the cell that the virus invades, the reverse
    transcriptase will cause the RNA to split and form
    the double-stranded DNA that the virus must have to
    reproduce. CDC illustration.

If such a material were found, it would have the
potential of eliminating viruses in the blood, but might
not affect the viruses already replicating in the T-4
cells. To stop virus reproduction, an agent would have
to be developed that could identify and selectively kill
the infected T-4 cells.

Given that the above reasoning is correct, it would
seem that two anti-AIDS agents are necessary, one to
attack the free virus in the blood and lymphatic system
and another to kill or neutralize the T-4 cells where the
virus is replicating. To expect one agent to tackle
these quite different tasks is asking a bit much, even
from the exciting world of biochemistry.

If the infected T-cells are not killed, it appears that a bit of genetic trickery is going to be needed to prevent reverse transcriptase activity and replication of the virus -- a biochemical block which would not allow DNA to form. Since these processes are taking place on a very small scale and include shared functions between the AIDS virus genes and the T-4 cell, attempting to stop reproduction of the virus within the cell will be difficult.

These two hypothetical agents, one to kill the free virus and another to naturalize the T-4 cells where the virus is reproducing, would potentially cure an infected person. It is too early to speculate what agent/s or approaches might be found to provide the best treatment for AIDS. A drug called suramin was thought in 1985 to block reverse transcriptase activity promise in vitro testing and prevent reproduction of the AIDS virus. Subsequent trials revealed that the drug was not effective in man in dosages that could be safely tolerated.

In the search for an anti-AIDS agent, many drugs will be eliminated because they are too toxic, have dangerous side effects, are ineffectual, must be perpetually administered, or cannot be made in sufficiently large quantities. The great majority of the drugs being tried will be eliminated for one or more of the above reasons, and then the choice will be made as to which of the remaining agents, or combinations of them, can be used for the safe, effective treatment of AIDS.

A vaccine is also needed to protected those who may be exposed to AIDS from becoming infected (21). The vaccine should be safe, of proven effectiveness, widely available, and inexpensive (22). This vaccine would induce the body to produce antibodies to the AIDS virus while not giving the person the disease.

The first vaccine ever administered was cowpox, used for inoculation against smallpox. After having the relatively mild cowpox, the body continued to produce antibodies which also protected a person against the deadly smallpox. This method worked because the cowpox antibody was similar enough to also protect against smallpox.

Another breakthrough came with the live virus vaccine for polio, where a weakened strain of the virus was used. Later the safer dead virus vaccine was developed. Rather than being the end of vaccine development, these steps led to using subunits of the infectious agent and genetically engineered or synthesized forms of these agents as a vaccine.

"Well, that doesn't seem so difficult. All you do is kill or injure a batch of the AIDS virus, inject them into somebody, and he is protected for life."

"O.K. fellow. Do you want the first shot?"

A major difficulty in developing a vaccine for the AIDS virus is that its external morphology differs from batch-to-batch of virus (23). Structurally, it's like trying to construct a building whose specifications keep changing. One month the owners decide they want cedar siding, the next marble slabs, the next half glass, and so on. A consistent, unique feature of the virus has to be found to use as a basis for vaccine development. The protecting agent must have something identifiable as a receptor site or it will not recognize the virus as the agent it is supposed to combat.

This genetic variation makes it difficult to design an AIDS vaccine. One approach, among others, that is now being used as a possible basis for vaccine development is stripping away the glycoprotein envelope of the virus, making batches of the envelope by using a hybridomas, a cancerous cell that can be "programmed" to reproduce particular proteins, and using the genetically inert viral envelope as a vaccine.

Injection of the viral envelope into a host would cause the host to make antibodies against the envelope. Then these antibodies would be available to fight off infections of the AIDS virus. However, if the AIDS virus differs in external structure, the antibodies would not recognize the infecting virus as the agent they were supposed to combat.

A point of hope is that a dead virus subunit vaccine has been developed for the retrovirus which causes feline leukemia, sometimes referred to as "AIDS in a cat."

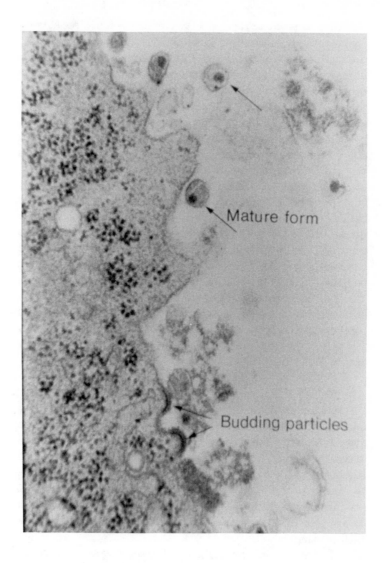

Figure 11. The HTLV-III virus budding and dispersing from
a giant multinucleated T-4 cell. The mature form of
the virus may circulate in the blood and lymphatic
system to infect other cells. CDC photo.

One science writer, Charles Seabrook of The Atlanta Constitution, summarized some of the approaches now being used to find a vaccine for AIDS. One is that the newly discovered HTLV-IV virus may be benign in humans, but could provide protection against the related HTLV-III virus. This approach is being investigated by Max Essex of Harvard University, among others. Another approach, by Gallo and others at the National Institutes of Health, is to remove genetic components from the HTLV-III virus so that a harmless virus results that would be similar enough to HTLV-III to be used as a vaccine (46).

Another investigation leading to a possible vaccine calls for inserting an AIDS-virus gene into the cowpox virus and determining if this hybrid virus can cause the body to produce sufficient numbers of AIDS antibodies to provide protection (46). Other workers are concentrating on the glycoprotein envelope of the virus, seeking to strip this protein away from the virus and using the entire protein shell as a possible vaccine or a conserved portion of the envelope that resists genetic change (46).

FROM CELL TO CELL

Once the virus enters the blood or lymphatic system, there is an opportunity to combat it before other cells are infected, but another problem in eliminating the virus is that it also infects the gray matter and fluid surrounding the brain (27). Any agent used to successfully combat AIDS must be able to cross the blood-central nervous-system boundary to destroy any virus that might be present in the nervous system that could reinfect the rest of the body.

In the brain, macrophage, or macrophage-like, cells are frequently isolated that have formed cancerous giant cells. Gallo speculates that these cells are the chief cause of lymphomas, lymphatic cancers of the brain. He also suggested that there may be an unidentified human retrovirus that targeted brain macrophage cells. He developed this line of reasoning because the genes of the

AIDS virus cannot be isolated from brain cancers (43).

Numerous researchers, Gallo among them, have isolated the AIDS virus from the brain. Gallo opinioned
that the virus in this case is carried in the cancerous
growths, but is apparently not the causative agent for
the cancers. If not the AIDS virus, then what? Another
retrovirus? Or, has the genetic material of the virus
been so altered or reintegrated in this type of cancer as
to be no longer recognizable?

It has been recognized, almost since the virus was
first identified, that isolates of the virus show great
genetic variation. These different isolates were first
thought to be geographically distributed and were described as Haitian, French, or New York isolates. Later
work revealed that not only did the isolates differ
according to geographic area, but they also differed in
the same individual over time (45).

Consideration was given to the possibility that
perhaps different isolates in the same person represented
different sources of infection. That one isolate was
introduced into the host during the first infection,
another variant on the second exposure, and so on; but
this hypothesis became untenable because similar variations were found in patients who had been continuously
hospitalized.

The observation that different isolates of the virus
could not be grown together in a culture also gave
evidence that competing AIDS viruses were not likely to
exist in the same host. In fact, thousands of generations of the AIDS virus can be grown in pure cultures
with very minor, if any, genetic variation (45).

Why the great differences occur in time in a human
host is incompletely understood, but Gallo postulated
that following infection by a particular strain of the
virus, say S1, this strain would mutate and make viral
variations S2-10. At one time strain S3 might be the
predominant strain, then perhaps S9, but, paradoxically,
strain S1 might again predominate. The agent that
prompts such wide genetic variations or the conditions
that might produce one strain of the virus rather than
another are not presently known.

FROM ANIMAL OR INSECT TO MAN

Central African green monkeys have a virus that is similar to the AIDS virus. Some Central African natives eat green monkeys. Some Central African natives have AIDS. Therefore, Central African natives contracted AIDS from green monkeys. The first three statements are true, but the conclusion is uncertain. It is possible that the disease was first introduced into man by someone butchering a green monkey, cutting his hand and absorbing the virus directly into the blood (24).

Such cross-species infections are not unusual in retroviruses, Gallo stated, and this is often the way in which a new pathologic organism may be introduced into a new host animal. The initial infection may have been a benign variant of the virus which may have caused no pathologic symptoms in man, but later through genetic variation developed its pathologic character (45).

The newly discovered human retroviruses, HTLV-IV and LAV 2, are closer in structure to the simian AIDS virus (SAV-III) than to the predominating AIDS virus in man (HTLV-III/LAV (HIV)).

The important point is not so much how the disease originated, but that a primate host exists for testing drugs and possible vaccines. Only the chimpanzee, an aggressive monkey poorly suited for a laboratory animal, will support an infection when exposed to the human AIDS virus. If chimps can be given a test AIDS vaccine, challenged with virus, and then successfully resist infection, this will open the way for vaccine trials in man. Because of the long incubation period of AIDS, such experiments will be time consuming. Test results in chimps must be examined carefully lest ambiguous results be interpreted as success and the political and economic pressures for early production of a vaccine result in the use of an ineffective agent.

Suspicion has fallen on mosquitos as being a possible transmission agent for the AIDS virus. This vector transmits malaria and yellow fever to man. So, why not AIDS too (28)?

In Belle Glade and Pahokee, Florida, Mark E. Whiteside found AIDS in 20 percent of a population (6 out of 29) with no other identifiable risk except exposure to environmental factors including the mosquitos Aedes aeqypti and Culex sp. and presented this data at the First International Conference on AIDS (29). A year later at the second international conference, Whiteside presented another poster identifying the presence of an arbovirus (a large group of viruses present in mosquitos, ticks, and mammals) in some AIDS patients (47).

This evidence only indicates that a person with AIDS had been bitten by mosquitos carrying the arbovirus and does not demonstrate that mosquitos carry the AIDS virus and are able to transmit it to man.

Jean-Claude Chermann of the Pasteur Institute released a report in the August, 1986, Proceedings of the Paris Academy of Sciences that most of a population group of 80 insects, mosquitos, cockroaches, ant-lions, and tsetse flies, from Zaire and the Central African Republic contained some fragments of the AIDS virus genes integrated into their genetic materials (48).

Chermann concluded, "The evidence from epidemiology is very clear that there is no way of (AIDS) transmission to humans by mosquitos or other insects." This opinion is also shared by other researchers in tropical medicine in Europe and the United States."

Nonetheless, a counter current of opinion persists among non-professional groups who continue to propagate the idea the mosquitos carry AIDS. Such a group was literally driven underground at the Second International Conference on AIDS and held an exhibit titled "Mosquitos DO Transmit AIDS" in the Paris Metro (subway) tunnel beneath the building where the conference was held.

Tabloid journalists find such information good copy for sensational treatment. The September 30, 1986, issue of Weekly World used Chermann's report as a basis for their story headlined "Household Pests Carry AIDS!" without including Chermann's statement that he considered it unlikely that the AIDS virus could be transmitted by insects to man (49).

An epidemiologic argument against the transmission of AIDS by mosquitos is that if mosquitos were carriers of AIDS, why isn't the disease much more widespread in areas like the southern United States than it is? There is a high prevalence of seropositivity in southern Florida and also a high prevalence of mosquitos. Why hasn't there been a much faster spread of AIDS among the "no-known-risk-factor group" up the Florida peninsula than has been observed? In cities like New York, San Francisco, or Los Angeles which also have mosquitos and large numbers of seropositive individuals, why hasn't there been a large increase of cases in the "no-known-risk-factor group?"

The great weight of scientific opinion and evidence is that mosquitos are not transmitters of AIDS to humans.

COFACTORS IN AIDS

There are no presently known cofactors that have been established that appear to: predetermine who will catch AIDS, how fast the disease will progress, explain why some people who have been exposed are not seropositive, or influence the survival time of a person with AIDS.

Several avenues have been explored, including use of poppers, histories of other sexually transmitted diseases, and exposure to agricultural chemicals with the result that except for the development of the "Safer Sex" recommendations, there has been no positive link established between possible cofactors and AIDS.

In the absence of being able to make a statement that this drug, that activity, or these foods will predispose one to or protect a seropositive individual from AIDS, general health care guidelines have been given. Basically these say avoid hazardous sexual activity, eat balanced meals, develop good sleep habits, avoid illegal drugs, drink in moderation, and stop smoking. The message is, "Take care of your body and it will probably do the best it can for you. Don't, and it can't."

Something that is important, but often ignored, is a person's mental state. If one is worried about the prospect of death, it is a bit too much to ask that he be concerned about whether or not he ate his spinach on Thursday. Some people need more support and services than others, but nearly all of those with AIDS will require nursing, social services, and household maintenance assistance during their illness. All of those providing these services are in a position to psychologically support those under their care or, if they cannot provide needed services, direct the person with AIDS to an appropriate person for counseling.

----

1. Centers for Disease Control, 1985, Update; acquired immunodeficiency syndrome - United States: Mortality Weekly Report, May 10.
2. Centers for Disease Control, 1986, United States: Mortality Weekly Report, May 26.
3. Centers for Disease Control, 1985, Revision of the case definition of acquired immunodeficiency syndrome for national reporting - United States: Mortality Weekly Report, June 28.
4. Centers for Disease Control, 1985, Update; revised public health service definition of persons who should refrain from donating blood and plasma - United States: Mortality Weekly Report, September 6.
5. Taylor, Ron, 1985, Paranoia over AIDS scaring blood donors away, Red Cross says: The Atlanta Constitution, October 10, 1985.
6. Centers for Disease Control, 1985, Update; Prospective evaluation of health-care workers exposed via the parenteral or mucous-membrane route to blood or body fluids from patients with acquired immunodeficiency syndrome - United States, Mortality Weekly Report, February 22.
6a. Seabrook, Charles, 1985, AIDS infects two working

with blood: The Atlanta Constitution, September 27.

7. Knight-Ridder Newspapers, 1985, Indiana town argues over boy's AIDS: The Atlanta Journal and Constitution, August 11.

8. Centers for Disease Control, 1985, Recommendations for preventing possible transmission of human T-cell lymphotrophic virus type III/lymphadeno-pathy-associated virus from tears: Mortality Weekly Report, August 30.

9. Centers for Disease Control, 1985, Update; Acquired immunodeficiency syndrome - United States: Mortality Weekly Report, May 10.

10. McKusick, Leon, 1985, Stability and change in gay sex; the case of San Francisco: Univ. California, San Francisco, and Univ. California, Berkeley, International Conference on AIDS, Atlanta, Georgia.

11. Anonymous, 1985, What gay and bisexual men should know about AIDS: Channing L. Bete Co, Inc., South Deerfield, Maryland.

12. Centers for Disease Control, 1985, Provisional public health service inter-agency recommendations for screening donated blood and plasma for antibody to the virus causing acquired immunodeficiency syndrome: Mortality Weekly Report, January 11.

13. Bay Area Physicians for Human Rights, 1984, AIDS safe-sex guidelines: San Francisco AIDS Foundation, San Francisco, California.

14. Howard Brown Memorial Clinic, 1983, AIDS patient information sheet: Howard Brown Memorial Clinic, Chicago, Illinois.

15. Anonymous, 1985, AIDS; A growing threat: Time Inc., New York, New York, August 12.

16. Harris, C.A., 1985, Immunodeficiency and HTLV-III/LAV serology in heterosexual partners of AIDS patients: Montefiore Medical Center, Bronx, New York; NCI, NIH, Bethesda, Maryland; and CDC, Atlanta; International Conference on AIDS, Atlanta, Georgia.

17. Callan, Monnie, 1985, Heterosexual AIDS patients and their Families; identification of psychosocial needs and provision of support services: Montefiore Medical Center, Albert Einstein College of Medicine, Bronx, New York; International Conference on AIDS, Atlanta, Georgia.

18. Ginzburg, Harold M., 1985, Educating parenteral drug users about AIDS: NIDA, ADAMHA, Rockville, Maryland, International Conference on AIDS, Atlanta, Georgia.

19. Clavel, Francois, 1985, The major glycoprotein of LAV (gp110); identification antigenicity and neutralizing capacity of specific antibodies: Pasteur Institute and La Pitie-Salpetriere Hospital, Paris, International Conference on AIDS, Atlanta, Georgia.

20. Popovic, Mikulas, 1985, Receptor mediated propagation of HTLV-III in human cells: NCI, NIH and Unif. Svcs. Univ. Hlth. Sciences, Bethesda, Maryland, International Conference on AIDS, Atlanta, Georgia.

21. Heckler, Margaret M., 1985, Keynote address: Secretary of health and human services, Washington, D.C., International Conference on AIDS, Atlanta, Georgia.

22. Annomyous, 1985, Vaccination for all Americans, The Atlanta Journal, April 16.

23. Levy, Jay, A., 1982, The clinical, biological and molecular features of AIDS-associated retroviruses (ARV): University of California, San Francisco, International Conference on AIDS, Atlanta, Georgia.

24. Gallo, Robert, C., 1985, The molecular biology and antigenic structure of HTLV-III: NCI, NIH, Bethesda, Maryland, International Conference on AIDS, Atlanta, Georgia.

25. Haseltine, William A., 1985, Transcriptional transactivation of the long terminal repeats of members of the HTLV-BLV retroviral family: Dana-Farber Cancer Inst., Boston, Massachu-

setts, and NCI, NIH, Bethesda, Maryland, International Conference on AIDS, Atlanta, Georgia.

26. Montagnier, Luc, 1985, Lymphadenopathy/AIDS virus; from molecular structure to pathogenicity: Viral Oncology Unit, Pasteur Institute, Paris, International Conference on AIDS, Atlanta, Georgia.

27. Jordan, B.D., 1985, Neurological complications of AIDS; an overview based on 110 autopsied patients: Cornell University Medical Center, New York City; Medical College New Jersey, Newark; and Memorial Sloan-Kettering Cancer Center, New York City, International Conference on AIDS, Atlanta, Georgia.

28. Thomas, Carroll, 1985, Reports; no evidence mosquitos carry AIDS: The Associated Press, Macon Telegraph and News, August 23.

29. Whiteside, Mark E., 1985, Outbreak of no-identifiable-risk acquired immunodeficiency syndrome in Belle Glade, Florida: Tropical Medicine, Miami, AIDS Program Manager HRS, Tallahassee; Palm Beach Health Department, Poster W-73, International Conference on AIDS, Atlanta, Georgia.

30. Volberding, P., 1986, Variation in AIDS-related illnesses; impact on clinical research: Second International Conference on AIDS, Paris, France.

31. National Public Radio, 1986, New recommendations on blood donations from National Institute of Health: Washington, D.C., July 17.

32. Madhok, R., 1986, Changes in factor use subsequent to publicity of AIDS in Haemophilia: Univ. Dept. of Medicine, Glasgow Royal Infirmary, Scotland, Second International Conference on AIDS, Paris, France.

33. Rosendaal, F.R., 1986, Attitude towards AIDS and the anti-LAV/HTLV-III test in Dutch Hemophiliacs: Dutch Hemophilia Society, Dept. of Hematology, University Hospital Leiden; Dept. of Medical Sociology, State University Groningen; Clinical

Genetics Centre Leiden; The Netherlands.

34. Gerberding, J. Louise, 1986, Risk of acquired immune deficiency syndrome (AIDS) virus transmission to health care workers; results of a prospective cohort study: Dept. of Medicine, Univ. of California, San Francisco and San Francisco General Hospital, San Francisco, California, U.S.A., Second International Conference on AIDS, Paris, France.

35. Griscelli, Claude, 1986, LAV-HTLV-III infection in infants and children: Dept. of Pediatrics, Hopital des Enfants Malades, Paris, France, Second International Conference on AIDS, Paris, France.

36. Rogers, Martha F., 1986, National surveillance for AIDS in children, United States: Centers for Disease Control, Atlanta, Second International Conference on AIDS, Paris, France.

37. Jaffee, Harold W., 1986, AIDS within population groups in the United States: Centers for Disease Control, Atlanta, Second International Conference on AIDS, Paris, France.

38. Conat, Marcus A., 1986, Condoms prevent transmission of the AIDS-associated retrovirus: Univ. of California in San Francisco, San Francisco, California, Second International Conference on AIDS, Paris, France.

39. Voeller, Bruce, 1986, Nonoxynol-9 and prevention of the sexual spread of LAV/HTLV-III and other STD agents: Mount Sinai School of Medicine, New York, Second International Conference on AIDS, Paris, France.

40. Mahler, H., 1986, World health organization's programme on AIDS: World Health Organization, Geneva, Switzerland, Second International Conference on AIDS, Paris, France.

41. Wofsy, Constance B., 1986, Isolation of AIDS associated retrovirus (ARV) from vaginal and cervical secretions of ARV seropositive women: Univ. of California, San Francisco, Second Interna-

tional Conference on AIDS, Paris, France.

42. Wijngaarden, Jan K. Van, 1986, AIDS policy co-ordination in the Netherlands: Polderweg 92, 1093 KP Amsterdam, the Netherlands.

43. Gallo, Robert C., 1986, Human retroviruses, now and in the future: National Institutes of Health, Bethesda, Maryland, U.S.A., Second International Conference on AIDS, Paris France.

44. Haseltine, William A., 1986, Structure and pathogenesis of the human T-Lymphotropic virus type III (HTLV-III/LAV): Dana-Farber Cancer Inst., Harvard Medical School, Boston, Mass. U.S.A., Second International Conference on AIDS, Paris, France.

45. Gallo, Robert C., 1986, Human retroviruses: National Institutes of Health, Bethesda, Maryland, U.S. A., 2nd World Congress on Sexually Transmitted Diseases, Paris, France.

46. Seabrook, Charles, 1986, Health authorities search feverishly for AIDS vaccine: The Atlanta Constitution, Atlanta, Georgia, U.S.A., August 4.

47. Whiteside, M. E., 1986, Arbovirus particles in the intestine of patients with acquired immunodeficiency syndrome (AIDS): Inst. of Tropical Medicine, Miami, Florida, Dept. of Pathology, Cedars Medical Center, Miami, Florida, U.S.A., Second International Conference on AIDS, Paris, France.

48. Spotnitz, Frank, 1986, Insects carrying AIDS are found in Africa: The Associated Press, in The Macon Telegraph and News, August 2.

49. Anonymous, 1986, Cockroaches carry AIDS: Weekly World News, September 30.

PREJUDICE AND PASSION

"Queers, drug addicts, and nigger immigrants. Those
are the people that have AIDS. I didn't have anything to
do with them before there was such a thing as AIDS, and I
sure as hell ain't going to do anything with them now."

The above would not be a comforting response to a
person who thought he might have AIDS and went to a
public health clinic. The prejudices and passions are
still there -- particularly in the more conservative
parts of the United States. Slowly, the information is
being disseminated even to the most thick-skulled that,
"AIDS is going to be around for a long time to come, and
you might as well get use to the idea."

A common series of events is that the person with
AIDS conceals his disease as long as possible to keep
from being fired from his job and losing his salary and
health benefits. Even if he is hospitalized, he tells
everyone he has cancer. When the word leaks out, or the
symptoms become obvious, he is informed that his job is
being eliminated as an economy measure and that even
though everyone will miss him very much, the company will
have to let him go.

His former friends, hearing of the news, drift away
and he becomes an isolated, social outcast. If he is
married, the wife and kids often pack up and move at
about this time.

He's jobless, friendless, familyless, probably nearly broke, and alone. Such a reversal of circumstances
might be expected to lead anyone into a state of depression and the contemplation of killing himself. This is
when the services provided by an AIDS support group are
desperately needed. Making contact with such a group
might not change his prognosis of survival, but being associated with those who understand what he is experi-
encing and being directed to where he can receive medical, psychological, financial, and social support will

certainly improve his quality of life.

Nearly every state has at least one agency to which AIDS patients can be referred. If one lived in an area where no such services were available, moving to a city where AIDS support groups were active might be appropriate. If such a move is contemplated, it should be within one's state of residence if at all possible because some state and locally-sponsored programs may be restricted to residents.

One case that received attention in the United States was that of Johnny Green, a 37-year-old writer who moved to New Orleans to take over the job of editing the in-house magazine of McDermott International Inc. (1). In the meantime, an article he wrote describing his personal fears that he might have AIDS was published in People Magazine. Four days after the magazine was stocked on the newsstands, Green received a notice that he was being fired because of "lack of productivity," even though he had recently submitted plans for the issues of the magazine through the following two years.

In fact, Green did not have AIDS. His only symptom was night sweats. He was seemingly fired on the basis of the suspicion that he might have the disease.

The same article quotes director Jim Kellogg, a member of the New York-based Lambda Defense Fund, a legal aid service, as stating, "The pattern in New Orleans and elsewhere is that you immediately lose your job when you appear to have either ARC or AIDS. Many times you lose your apartment and also your health insurance. Nobody in their right mind would proclaim they are gay and then try to find a job right now."

Johnny Green? He's back free-lancing magazine articles for Town and Country, Playboy and Harper's. As of July, 1985, he still did not have AIDS.

In New York, the Rev. Kenneth J. Smith, a parish priest, criticized the members of his parish for opposing a shelter for those with AIDS stating, "The weakest of our community need help, and we were unable to offer that help (2).

"As a priest who has been preaching the Gospel for

many years, I am somewhat saddened by the attitude of rejection," Smith told the members of the Holy Name of Jesus Church who opposed using an abandoned convent as a shelter for AIDS patients. The convent building is adjacent to a church school, and most of the opposition was from parents whose children attended the school. Their opposition led to the cancellation of the plans for the shelter by the Roman Catholic Archdiocese of New York.

Some parishioners supported their priest and were represented in the news article as having said that the Holy Name church had sponsored programs for alcoholics, drug addicts, and the homeless, and the AIDS shelter was just an extension of these programs.

Discrimination against an individual and against a group of parishioners is repugnant; but even a national ethnic group, the Haitians, have also been subjected to a great deal of pressure since they were the only identifiable ethnic group mentioned by the CDC in connection with AIDS.

A Miami newspaper article states their plight as being considered carriers of the disease with the result that wide-spread psychological, financial, and social damage has resulted from this group's linkage with AIDS (3). The CDC has since dropped Haitians as a group listing in its reports.

Nonetheless, damage has been done with the results that Haitians are still being denied jobs, apartments, and deprived of social contacts among school children that would have otherwise occurred over the past four years. This group has been stigmatized even though the majority of Haitians have not been exposed to AIDS.

There are some signs of hope. The advertising campaign, "L.A. Cares Like A Mother," and others like it are indications that some of the social stigmatization associated with first being gay or a Haitian and secondly, having AIDS, is slowly being removed. Still, problems about fairness in employment, housing, and medical treatment persist.

The most difficult group to reach are IV drug users. Particular services are being designed at some national drug abuse clinics to assist those users willing to be helped.

Hemophiliacs and others who contracted AIDS through blood transfusions or contaminated blood products are also being subjected to discrimination because of the strong association in most people's minds that a person with AIDS is gay. It is often trauma enough to be identified as gay if one is, but to be identified as gay and not be gay adds an additional psychological burden to those who have transfusion-caused AIDS. For children in this category, the mental burden is particularly difficult to deal with.

HOMOPHOBIA

Homophobia means "fear of homosexuals." While such a fear may be held by some individuals at about the same frequency as others are terrified of spiders, the word probably more nearly relates to feelings of disgust or repugnance at the thought of man-to-man or woman-to-woman sexual activity. Often, the picture a person has in his mind is of a child abuser or a guy dressed in an outrageous drag costume. There are individuals who fit this description who are homosexuals, but there are also the great majority of homosexuals and bisexuals that one would never recognize from their appearance or actions. They are as individualistic as anyone, and they do not fit these or other stereotypes.

Many bisexuals are married, and they and their families live out their lives in an identical fashion with their neighbors, except that the husband may occasionally also engage in gay sexual activity or have done so in the past. It is by no means impossible that he might remain completely faithful to his wife.

There are monogamous homosexual couples who have lived together for years and consider themselves "married." On occasion, vows are exchanged; and although this may seem to some a perversion of religion, these vows serve as a public notice that this couple is married and they have pledged themselves to remain true to each other throughout their lives. Such a "marriage" has no legal standing under state laws. For one member of such a marriage to protect his interest, detailed wills must be drawn to insure that any joint estate (or in many cases the other partner's property) is properly divided after the death of one partner.

Solitary homosexuals who have no wish to be drawn into a long-term relationship or who have not found an acceptable partner, or are between partners, form the majority of the homosexual population. In San Francisco single homosexuals were found to be about 58 percent of the gay population with 42 percent reporting that they are in a monogamous relationship (4). This large percentage of the gay population as well as that portion in monogamous relationships that allow outside sexual activity are the groups having the highest risk for AIDS.

In the San Francisco business world, a person would find it difficult to determine who was gay and who was not. The waiter escorting you to the table might be gay, or the bartender, or that businessman at the next table closing a million-dollar real estate transaction, or the lawyer-looking type grabbing a sandwich at the bar between court appearances, or the busboy who's clearing the table -- men indistinguishable from thousands of others that one might see in a city on a busy day.

Are the health needs of such people worthy of concern? This is a question that each person who might deal with the health care of gays must honestly answer. If the answer is negative, if there is no understanding by health care personnel of the problems of caring for gay patients, then reluctant care providers should seek work in another area of the health profession (5).

A poster presented at the Second International Conference on AIDS sought to examine the attitudes of health-care professionals about caring for AIDS patients. Thomas P. Kalman of Cornell University polliing a population of 128 doctors and nurses found that the average ranking in the study demonstrated a "low-grade homophobic range...with women being more homophobic than men a contrast with all previous studies." One finding which Kalman categorized as alarming was that 10 percent of those tested thought that, "Homosexuals who contract AIDS are getting what they deserved (12).

Fred Gordon of the Veterans Administration Medical Center in Washington, D.C., presented a presentation based on a study of 1194 hospital workers to determine their attitudes towards caring for AIDS patients at the second international conference. His findings were that most health workers surveyed had strong reservations about caring for AIDS patients with 25 percent expressing extreme anxiety, and more than half were misinformed about needed precautions (thinking that gowns and masks were necessary for every care administration) (13).

Gordon concluded, "This study documents suboptimal knowledge about and behavior towards AIDS patients and suggests that in-service education and counseling which provides accurate knowledge about AIDS may result in less anxiety and more compassionate and appropriate patient care."

Gay patients are not asking that the care provider condone gayness or become gay, just to accept that a gay is entitled to the same level of health care and compassion as anyone else facing a potentially fatal illness.

Additional factors are that a gay's family may not be his biological family and a gay couple's relationship is just as deep as a heterosexual couple's. Visiting rights in intensive care wards and the counseling that would be given a spouse and family should be extended to the other partner and close friends in a gay relationship (5). Both the one who is ill and his lover have deep psychological concerns over the outcome of the disease and the prognosis for survival. The member of the pair who is not being hospitalized carries with him the added burden of knowing that he has been exposed to AIDS and must watch and wait for the "time bomb" to go off and the first symptoms to appear.

He may be lucky, he may never have AIDS, or the onset of symptoms may be delayed for years. In the meantime, he should be informed that he is potentially

infectious and should avoid unsafe and questionably safe
sex practices until such a time that a cure is found.

These are the sort of caring concerns that must be
administered in health care.

The business world in the United States has not
been   much concerned with the health and well-being of
its employees.   Health plans have been, and are being,
offered by most of the larger businesses as an employee
incentive; but to say that management cares deeply about
the health of its workers is more loose words than fact.
If management had a suspicion that a person had AIDS,
ARC, had tested positively for the AIDS virus or was gay,
more times than not some means would be found for the
rapid dismissal of that employee -- typically with a loss
of health benefits as well as salary.

A person should be allowed to work for as long as he
is able; when he becomes unable to work, be allowed to
withdraw from his job with at least six months' health
insurance benefits intact.

Another business-related problem arises when an
application is made for a job. What about when the
questions: "Do you now have or have you ever had AIDS or
ARC, or received a positive test for the AIDS virus?
Will you take a lie detector test to verify the above
answer?" start appearing on the nation's job application
forms?   The above is so obviously discriminatory that
more   subtle questions such as "Have you undergone any
test by a health care provider, been hospitalized, or
been treated for an immunodeficiency disease during the
past five years?" are now being used on employment and
insurance forms. Unless legal action is taken to prevent
this information from being released as a violation of a
basic right to privacy, such questions would effectively
bar many gays from jobs.

For this reason and out of fear that confidiality
will be breached, many gays have refused to take the
ELISA blood test to determine if they have been infected
with the AIDS virus (6). Once identified as being infected or as being gay, they fear losing their jobs, increases or cancellations of insurance policies, lease

cancellations, or other adverse effects on their lives.

The United States Army has now instituted ELISA test screening of all new recruits and members of the army with the justification that in a battlefield situation, any soldier might be called upon to give a transfusion to a wounded individual, and to place the wounded soldier in jeopardy of an AIDS infection is unjustified (7).

In cases where a recruit gives a seropositive test, he is not allowed to join the army. In the event that a person on active duty or in the reserves is found to give a seropositive test, and this test is confirmed, present practice is often to dismiss that person from the service with resulting loss of accrued retirement and health benefits or place him into a non-combat role.

Deep reservations have been expressed by civil rights organizations and psycosocial service providers as to the legality of universally administering the test to those who are forced to take it, about preserving the confidentiality of test results, and the present lack of counseling offered to those, recruits and active duty personnel alike, who may have a seropositive result.

Homosexual acts, under the Uniform Code of Military Justice, which applies to all armed forces of the United States, are court martial offenses and subject any individual convicted of committing a penetrative act to the possibility of a dishonorable discharge. Standards were relaxed during the Vietnam War, and a claim of homosexuality would not prevent a person from being drafted if he was otherwise qualified for service. During the war and after it, homosexuals have been admitted to the nation's armed forces and comprise an unknown percentage of the services' populations.

These circumstances put the homosexual serviceman in a quandary. If he admits to being a homosexual, he may be discharged from the service. If he cannot say that he is a homosexual, how does he avoid giving blood when the pressure is on for a unit to make the 100 percent mark in blood donations? An appropriate answer is to say that he has had hepatitis and has been advised never to give blood. What if he comes down with ARC or AIDS? The only assertion that he can make without possibly losing health care benefits is to say that he was infected by a prostitute. There is no official military stigma attached to to the contraction of venereal diseases, so long as these diseases are promptly reported and treated -- this is not a military offense, but the homosexual contraction of AIDS may be.

Because of the implied threat of punishment, the admission of homosexual activity by a serviceman would be unusual, and reports of servicemen contracting AIDS through relations with prostitutes are suspect.

Unless prevented by legal action, ELISA testing of blood samples could be made a part of a pre-employment physical administered to a prospective employee. The United States Army has paved the way for the adoption of this screening technique by industry. The results of ELISA test are only conclusive if they are positive. A negative test does not necessarily mean that the person's blood is free of the virus -- only that no detectable antibodies to the virus were found. The test is not 100 percent reliable and a few percentages of false reports do occur. When a positive result is returned, it is tested again by the ELISA method, and confirmed by another test, such as the Western Blot.

Social deprivation and isolation from friends and family are two of the most crushing blows that can be administered to a person with AIDS. Relationships that have been developed over many years suddenly become cold. Friends scurry away when approached, children are rushed inside the house, people talk through doors -- it is as if a Biblical leper was suddenly dropped down on suburban America.

One cannot control the thoughts of others, but at least a person can inform his friends and family and quiet some of their fears about AIDS. This is a heavy trip, and it is best done with the assistance of a sympathetic doctor. The fair-weather friends will fall by the way, but those that remain will be able to assist one through any coming crises.

Membership in churches and social organizations does

not count for much once a person has been diagnosed with AIDS. These will most often effectively shun an individual or treat him in such a manner that it becomes more of a pain than a supporting function to attend church services or to go to meetings. To those who have led an active community life, this is a serious deprivation and a shock to find that lodge members, "sworn ever to be faithful to each other," have added the corollary, "except when one of us has AIDS."

Gay organizations in the larger cities offer some means of regaining an active social life through conference groups and activities as well as providing information and services. There are also gay church groups that provide religious as well as social support to those with AIDS.

Not all the news is negative. Los Angeles has passed an ordinance protecting those with AIDS from discrimination in employment, housing, and health care (9). San Francisco General Hospital has in place a system of health care for AIDS patients that provides for counseling, in-hospital care, and community support of AIDS patients (5). The approaches applied to the treatment of AIDS patients at the hospital have been widely used as a model by other American hospitals. States in which relatively few AIDS cases have been reported have begun to recognize the seriousness and permanence of the AIDS problem and have plans to prepare for increasing numbers of AIDS patients and their psychosocial problems (10).

FAMILY CONSIDERATIONS

Telling a present or former wife that one has AIDS and that she may have been infected with the virus is a traumatic experience, particularly if the man had managed to keep his homosexual experiences from her for a period of years. This would come as an unexpected, crushing blow that might lead to a sense of non-believing numbness, violent outburst, recriminations, and possibly the break up of the marriage.

If such a condition should exist, it must be faced and dealt with, because future penetrative sexual contact must be avoided or protective measures taken during sex. The wife and children should also be tested to determine if they are infected with the virus so that, again, proper and prudent precautions can be taken.

Unlike herpes where a child can often be spared the infection by being delivered by cesarean section, AIDS can infect the child in the womb as well as during birth. Studies are now in progress to attempt to determine the risks of pregnancy, but no conclusive recommendations have been reached. Any woman who has had sexual relations with either bisexuals or IV drug users or who has had a large number of sexual partners should be tested for AIDS antibodies prior to considering pregnancy, according to present CDC recommendations (8).

Once pregnancy occurs, there is no readily accessible way to predict if the child will subsequently develop AIDS. Some children born to AIDS antibody positive mothers do develop AIDS, but others may test positively for the AIDS antibody for only a few weeks after birth, and later give a negative antibody test and no indications of infection (14).

What is the risk that a child born to an antibody positive mother will develop AIDS?

In an article on Claude Griselli printed in the French newspaper Liberation published on June 24, 1986, Gilles Pial reported a study done in the Hospital of Childhood Diseases in Paris. The newspaper article stated that 56 women who were seropositive, 75 percent of them heroin users, gave birth (15). In following these children Griselli reported during the Second International Conference on AIDS that children who remained without symptoms of immune deficiency from four to six months after birth were rare, that 60 percent developed signs of immune deficiency, and that 30 percent developed AIDS (16). Griselli concluded, "The high proportion of severe forms of HTLV-III/LAV infection in infants and the modest effect of therapy tend to justify proposition of contraception and raise the delicate question of abortion at the beginning of pregnancy for seropositive women (16)."

A group of five pregnant women who were seropositive gave birth at the Montefiore Medical Center in New York. All five had full-term live births, there were no prenatal complications, and none of the children developed AIDS-related illnesses one-to-four months after delivery according to Peter A. Selwyn of the hospital (17).

Kataka Tshibangu of the Department of Obstetrics at the University of Kinshasa in Zaire reported case studies of five pregnant women with chronic diarrhea which lasted from 3-to-18 months. In two cases the fetuses died, in two cases the babies died at birth, and in the fifth case the infant failed to thrive and died, probably of AIDS, after living 12 months. He concluded that the clinical course of AIDS in the mothers worsened with pregnancy and suggested that pregnancy may accelerate the onset of fatal illness (18).

These three studies point out unresolved contradictions about the risks to a expectant seropositive mother and her unborn child. The transient seropositivity observed in some children born by seropositive mothers would appear to partially negate the approach of testing fetal blood for AIDS antibodies because some fetuses would test positively but, if brought to full term might never exhibit AIDS-related symptoms.

The above assumes that the fetus was infected in the womb, as Tshibangu's results would seem to indicate.

The reasons why 100 percent of the seropositive mothers in Selwyn's group were able to give birth without apparently passing on the virus to their children while 90 percent of the children born to seropositive mothers in Griselli's work did develop AIDS-related symptoms is unknown.

Pregnancy risk determination remains another of the problems of AIDS to which there is, as yet, no clear-cut answer.

Casual contact in a family setting, even when more than one family member has AIDS, has not been demonstrated to be a method of transmitting AIDS to other members of the family (8).

SOCIAL NEEDS

A general consensus of the First International Conference on AIDS was that the scientific knowledge of the disease was advancing more rapidly than the development of social services for AIDS and ARC patients and the larger population of "worried well." This disease, more than any that man has seen, is very intensive in its requirements for disseminating of information, counseling patients and their families as well as the "worried well," providing in-home care and support for AIDS patients, giving financial support for the families of those with AIDS, and replacing out-dated information as quickly as possible.

The proper design and administration of these programs must be done with the knowledge that many popularly held stereotypes about gays and others with AIDS are not true. There are, for example, gays who have wives and children; Hispanic gays, black gays, and oriental gays; users of IV drugs who are not addicts; and an increasingly large percentage of those with AIDS in the United States who are in minority groups, not well educated, and live below the poverty level.

A July 22, 1986, Associated Press article quoted Wayne Greaves, chief of infection control at Howard University Hospital in Washington, D.C., as observing black women account for 52 percent of all female cases of AIDS, and black children, 60 percent of AIDS cases in their age group. "With blacks representing only 12 percent of the United States population, these are serious numbers (19)."

The same article, referring to testing of military recruits, stated that an early June, 1986, CDC analysis of this data demonstrated that among this population group the seropositivity rate of blacks was four times that of whites (20).

Now that the scope and duration of the fight against AIDS is clearly seen as involving the entire world in a battle against the syndrome that will last well into the 21st century, developing effective psychosocial support programs for those who have AIDS becomes increasingly important. The survival time for those who have AIDS is also increasing because of advances being made towards treating and defeating opportunistic infections. Again, there will be an even larger population of individuals who will need psychosocial support as well as in-home medical care.

The challenges that AIDS presents in the field of social services are no less demanding than those that are facing medical science -- challenges that in many parts of the United States remain unmet.

Rock Hudson's admission that he had AIDS and his death on October 2, 1985, focused a great deal of public attention on the disease. If Hudson was gay or not, and how or when he contracted the disease, is of little importance compared to the galvanizing effect on the public that a well-known figure had AIDS. The last public statement issued by Hudson was read by Burt Lancaster at a celebrity benefit to raise money to for AIDS research.

"I am not happy that I am sick," the statement said. "I am not happy that I have AIDS. But if that is helping others, I can at least know that my own misfortune has had some positive worth."

It is ironic that Hudson will be more rembered as the person who "brought AIDS out of the closet" rather than for a long, successful acting career. Knowingly or not and willingly or not, Hudson did more to overcome the stigma attached to the disease than any other person -- an unusual legacy, but a welcome one.

----

1. Cawthon, Raad, 1985, Fired after AIDS article, writer fears bias on rise: The Atlanta Journal-Constitution, July 21, 1985.
2. Anonymous, 1985, N.Y. priest criticizes parish for rejecting AIDS victims: The New York Times, Atlanta Journal-Constitution, September 2.

3. McCarthy, Kathy, 1985, Haitians; Taking us off AIDS list can't lift stigma: The Miami Herald, April 11.

4. Shilts, Randy, 1984, 70,000 gay men in San Francisco, first big study says: The San Francisco Chronicle, November 15.

5. Volderding, Paul A., 1985, Clinical Manifestations of AIDS: San Francisco General Hospital and University of California, San Francisco, International Conference on AIDS, Atlanta, Georgia.

6. Haithman, Diane, 1985, Fear undermining effectiveness of AIDS test, research groups say: Knight-Ridder Newspapers, Macon Telegraph and News, August 24.

7. Black, Norman, 1985, AIDS test ordered for all recruits: The Associated Press, Macon Telegraph and News, August 31.

8. Centers for Disease Control, 1985, Provisional public health inter-agency recommendations for screening donated blood and plasma for antibody to the virus causing acquired immunodeficiency syndrome: Mortality Weekly Report, January 11.

9. Anonymous, 1985, LA bans discrimination against AIDS victims: The Atlanta Constitution, August 15.

10. Galloway, Jim, 1985, State forms task force on AIDS: The Atlanta Constitution, September 19.

11. Lyman, Rick, 1985, Hudson loses AIDS battle, dies in sleep: Macon Telegraph and News, October 3.

12. Kalman, Thomas P., 1986, Homophobia among physicians and nurses; an empirical study: Cornell Univ. Medical College (Dept. of Psychiatry), New York, U.S.A., Second International Conference on AIDS, Paris, France.

13. Gordin, Fred, 1986, Hospital workers' knowledge, behavior and attitudes towards AIDS: Veterans Administration Medical Center, Washington, D.C., and National Institutes of Health, Bethesda, Maryland, U.S.A., Second International Conference on AIDS, Paris, France.

14. Fischel, M. A., 1986, Heterosexual and household

transmission of the human T-lymphotrophic virus type III: Univ. of Miami School of Medicine, Miami, Florida, U.S.A., Second International Conference on AIDS, Paris, France.

15. Pial, Gilles, 1986, L'enigme des bebes du SIDA: Liberation, Paris, France, June 24.

16. Griscelli, Claude, LAV-HTLV-III infection in infants and children: Dept: of Pediatrics, Hopital des Enfants Malades, Paris, France, Second International Conference on AIDS, Paris, France.

17. Selwyn, Peter, A., 1986, HTLV-III/LAV infection and pregnancy outcomes in intravenous drug abusers: Montefiore Medical Center, Albert Einstein College of Medicine, Bronx, New York, U.S.A., Second International Conference on AIDS, Paris, France.

18. Tshibangu, Kataka, 1986, Personal communication: Dept. of Obstetrics, Univ. of Zaire, Second International Conference on AIDS, Paris, France, June 23.

19. Associated Press, 1986, Tests by military indicate blach recruits' AIDS rate exceeds whites' four times: The Associated Press, in The Macon Telegraph and News, July 22.

20. Centers for Disease Control, 1986, HTLV-III/LAV antibody prevalence in U.S. military recruit applicants: Mortality Weekly Report, Centers for Disease Control, Atlanta, Georgia, U.S.A., July 4.

PRECAUTIONS FOR HEALTH WORKERS

FOR THE ORDINARY CARE of a mentally competent AIDS patient special precautions are required to prevent infection of health-care personnel, but the precautions recommended by the United States Public Health Service are little different from those advised for the treatment of patients with hepatitis B (1). No high-cost items of special equipment are needed for the care of AIDS patients in a typical hospital. Most of the recommendations concern preventing the transfer of the AIDS virus by the use of protective clothing, the disposal of body products, and the discard or sterilization of instruments.

Treating a typical AIDS patient would not require special gowns, shoe coverings, goggles, masks, gloves or a "moon suit" to protect the health care provider, although gloves should be worn when handling body waste products, blood-stained waste, tissue samples, and, by inference, when bathing a patient (1).

A listing of precautions to be observed by clinical and laboratory staffs is given in a six-page booklet published by the health service which contains three reprinted articles from the Centers for Disease Control morbidity and mortality weekly reports. The article relating to clinical and laboratory precautions first appeared in the Weekly Mortality Report of November 5, 1982, and has since been expanded by the CDC (1).

The recommended precautions are listed below:

PATIENT CARE

A. The following precautions are advised in providing care to AIDS patients;

    1. Extraordinary care must be taken to avoid accidental wounds from sharp instruments contaminated with potentially infectious material and to avoid contact of open skin lesions with material from AIDS

patients.

2.   Gloves should be worn when handling blood specimens, blood-soiled items, body fluids, excretions,
and secretions, as well as surfaces, materials, and
objects exposed to them.

3.   Gowns should be worn when clothing may be soiled
with body fluids, blood, secretions, or excretions.

4.   Hands should be washed after removing gowns and
gloves and before leaving the rooms of known or
suspected AIDS patients. Hands should also be washed
thoroughly and immediately if they become contaminated with blood.

5.   Blood and other specimens should be labeled
prominently with a special warning, such as "Blood
Precautions" or "AIDS Precautions." If the outside
of the specimen container is visibly contaminated
with blood, it should be cleaned with a disinfectant
(such as 1:10 dilution of 5.25% sodium hypochlorite
(household bleach) with water). All blood specimens
should be placed in a second container, such as an
impervious bag, for transport. This container or bag
should be examined carefully for leaks or cracks.

6.   Blood spills should be cleaned up promptly with
a disinfectant solution, such as sodium hypochlorite.

7.   Articles soiled with blood should be placed in
an impervious bag prominently labeled "AIDS Precautions" or "Blood Precautions" before being sent for
reprocessing or disposal. Alternatively, such contaminated items may be placed in plastic bags of a
particular color designated solely for disposal in
accord with the hospital's policies for disposal of
infectious wastes. Reusable items should be repro-
cessed in accord with hospital policies for hepatitis
B virus-contaminated items. Lensed instruments
should be sterilized after use on AIDS patients.

8.   Needles should not be bent after use, but should
be promptly placed in a puncture-resistant container
used solely for such disposal. Needles should not be
reinserted into their original sheaths before being
discarded into the container, since this is a common

cause of needle injury.

9.   Disposable syringes and needles are preferred.
Only needle-locking syringes or one-piece needle-
syringe units should be used to aspirate fluids from
patients so that collected fluid can be safely discharged through the needle, if desired. If reusable
syringes are employed, they should be decontaminated
before reprocessing.

10.   A private room is indicated for patients who
are too ill to use good hygiene, such as those with
profuse diarrhea, fecal incontinence, or altered
behavior secondary to central nervous system infections.

Precautions appropriate for particular infections
that concurrently occur in AIDS patients should be
added to the above, if needed.

These care guidelines are explicit in some details,
but not in others.   The question of how a patient is to
be bathed, presuming that he is unable to bathe himself,
is not specifically answered.   From number 2 above, it
would appear that gloves should be worn since the
patient's skin is certainly a surface exposed to blood,
body fluids, excretions, and secretions.

In relating these guidelines to a home care setting,
the use of gloves, tough plastic bags, quantities of
diluted bleach solutions for cleaning spills on floors,
etc., washing any cloth item that the patient has used
in separate loads with bleach would appear to be steps
that could be taken to protect other family members from
infection. Casual contact between family members has not
been demonstrated as being a transmission path for AIDS,
but it is reasonable to avoid skin contact with any
sores that the patient may have or with any of the patient's body products or items soiled by them.

The health service recommendations continue (1):

LABORATORY PRECAUTIONS

B. The following precautions are advised for persons performing laboratory tests or studies on clinical specimens or other potentially infectious materials (such as inoculated tissue cultures, embryonated eggs, animal tissues, etc.) from known or suspected AIDS cases.

1. Mechanical pipetting devices should be used for the manipulation of all liquids in the laboratory. Mouth pipetting should not be allowed.

2. Needles and syringes should be handled as stipulated in Section A (above).

3. Laboratory coats, gowns, or uniforms should be worn while working with potentially infectious materials and should be discarded appropriately before leaving the laboratory.

4. Gloves should be worn to avoid skin contact with blood, specimens containing blood, blood-soiled items, body fluids, excretions, and secretions, as well as surfaces, materials, and objects exposed to them.

5. All procedures and manipulations of potentially infectious material should be performed carefully to minimize the creation of droplets and aerosols.

6. Biological safety cabinets (Class I or II) and other primary containment devices (e.g., centrifuge safety cups) are advised whenever procedures are conducted that have a high potential for creating aerosols or infectious droplets. These include centrifuging, blending, sonicating, vigorous mixing, and harvesting infected tissues from animals or embryonated eggs. Fluorescent activated cell sorters generate droplets that could potentially result in infectious aerosols. Translucent plastic shielding between the droplet-collecting area and the equipment operator should be used to reduce the presently uncertain magnitude of this risk. Primary containment devices are also used in handling materials that might contain concentrated infectious

agents or organisms in greater quantities than expected in clinical specimens.

7. Laboratory work surfaces should be decontaminated with a disinfectant, such as sodium hypochlorite solution (see A5 above), following any spill of potentially infectious material and the completion of work activities.

8. All potentially contaminated materials used in laboratory tests should be decontaminated, preferably by autoclaving, before disposal or reprocessing.

9. All personnel should wash their hands following completion of laboratory activities, removal of protective clothing, and before leaving the laboratory.

Although the aerosol droplets mentioned above were those that might be caused by accidents in a laboratory setting, the droplets given off by a patient's sneeze may sometimes fall into the same category. A patient prone to sneezing or coughing episodes is inadvertently releasing droplets of mucosal material into the air. In the limited case where a patient is suffering from a respiratory infection that might be transmitted to other patients, and not just an opportunistic infection like KS confined to the skin, it would appear appropriate to mask and gown before entering that patient's room. The patient should be informed why these precautions are necessary in his case, but seeing all AIDS patients while wearing masks and gowns should not be done on a routine basis because of the additional psychological and social alienation that these measures give to the patient.

Experimental Animals

C. The following additional precautions are advised for studies involving experimental animals inoculated with tissues or other potentially infectious materials from individuals with known or suspected

AIDS.

1. Laboratory coats, gowns, or uniforms should be worn by personnel entering rooms housing inoculated animals. Certain nonhuman primates, such as chimpanzees, are prone to throw excreta and to spit at attendants; personnel attending inoculated animals should wear molded surgical masks and goggles or other equipment sufficient to prevent potentially infective droplets from reaching the mucosal surfaces of their mouths, nares (noses), and eyes. In addition, when handled, other animals may disturb excreta in their bedding. Therefore, the above precautions should be taken when handling them.

2. Personnel should wear gloves for all activities involving direct contact with experimental animals and their bedding and cages. Such manipulations should be performed carefully to minimize the creation of aerosols and droplets.

3. Necropsy of experimental animals should be conducted by personnel wearing gowns and gloves. If procedures generating aerosols are performed, masks and goggles should be worn.

4. Extraordinary care must be taken to avoid accidental sticks or cuts with sharp instruments contaminated with body fluids or tissues of experimental animals inoculated with material from AIDS patients.

5. Animal cages should be decontaminated, preferably by autoclaving, before they are cleaned and washed.

6. Only needle-locking syringes or one-piece needle-syringe units should be used to inject potentially infectious fluids into experimental animals.

The above precautions are intended to apply to both clinical and research laboratories. Biological safety cabinets and other safety equipment may not be generally available in clinical laboratories. Assistance should be sought from a microbiology laboratory, as needed, to assure containment facilities are adequate to permit laboratory tests to be conducted safely.

The precautions in regard to dress outlined in C1 would also appear to be applicable to humans who, either by reasons of hostility or because of mental disease, display similar aggression towards those caring for them.

SURGICAL PROCEDURES

Seeing the need for more detailed recommendations the CDC issued on April 11, 1986, "Recommendations for Preventing Transmission of Infection with Human T-Lymphotropic Virus Type III/Lymphadenopathy-Associated Virus during Invasive Procedures." These recommendations were intended for physicians, nurses, dentists, and others who might assist in a surgical procedure. The eight recommendations follow (4):

1. All HCWs (health-care workers) who perform or assist in operative, obstetric, or dental invasive procedures must be educated regarding the epidemiology, modes of transmission, and prevention of HTLV-III/LAV infection and the need for routine use of appropriate barrier precautions during procedures and when handling instruments contaminated with blood after procedures.

2. All HCWs who perform or assist in invasive procedures must wear gloves when touching mucous membranes or nonintact skin of all patients and use other appropriate barrier precautions when indicated (e.g. masks, eye coverings, and gowns, if aerosolization or splashes are likely to occur). In the dental setting, as in the operative and obstetric setting, gloves must be worn for touching all mucous membranes and changed between all patient contacts. If a glove is torn or a needlestick or other injury occurs, the glove must be changed as promptly as safety permits and the needle or instrument removed from the sterile field.

3.   All HCWs who perform or assist in vaginal or cesarean deliveries must use appropriate barrier precautions (e.g. gloves and gowns) when handling the placenta or the infant until blood and amniotic fluid have been removed from the infant's skin.

4.   All HCWs who perform or assist in invasive procedures must use extraordinary care to prevent injuries to hands caused by needles and other sharp instruments during procedures; when cleaning used instruments; during disposal of used needles; and when handling sharp instruments following procedures. After use, disposable syringes and needles, scalpel blades, and other sharp items must be placed in puncture-resistant containers for disposal. To prevent needlestick injuries, needles should not be recapped; purposefully bent or broken; removed from disposable syringes; or otherwise manipulated by hand.

5.   If an incident occurs during an invasive procedure that results in exposure of a patient to the blood of an HCW, the patient should be informed of the incident, and previous recommendations for management of such exposures (MMWR 1985;34:682-6,691-5) followed.

6.   No HCW who has exudative lesions or weeping dermatitis should perform or assist in invasive procedures or other direct patient-care activities or handle equipment used for patient care.

7.   All HCWs with evidence of any illness that may compromise their ability to adequately and safely perform invasive procedures should be evaluated medically to determine whether they are physically and mentally competent to perform invasive procedures.

8.   Routine serologic testing for evidence of HTLV-III/LAV infection is not necessary for HCWs who perform or assist in invasive procedures or for patients undergoing invasive procedures, since the risk of transmission in this setting is so low. Results of such routine testing would not practically

supplement the precautions recommended above in further reducing the negligible risk of transmission during operative, obstetric, or dental invasive procedures.

The above recommendations are obviously intended to prevent the possible transmission of AIDS from the patient to the health-care worker or from the health-care worker to the patient. An important aspect of the recommendations is that routine serologic testing, either of the patient or the health-care worker, is not recommended. Instead, strict precautionary measures are advocated instead of routine testing which many health-care workers and patients would find offensive. For serologic testing to provide a degree of protection, testing of health care workers would have to be done at not less than monthly intervals, or perhaps even weekly, which would be burdensome to health care workers and hospitals. The alternative of testing patients when they enter the hospital would draw strong protest if health care workers were not also subjected to testing.

DENTAL-CARE PERSONNEL

While not in quite as high a level of risk as other health-care professionals who routinely perform invasive surgical procedures, preventing the transmission of AIDS and other diseases from the patient to the dental care provider and from the care provider to the patient is recognized by the CDC as being an important concern.

An article published on April 18, 1986, by the CDC amplifies previous, more general, precautions issued on November 5, 1982, in which the following recommendations appeared (1, 5):

1. Personnel should wear gloves, masks, and protective eyewear when performing dental or oral surgical procedures.

2. Instruments used in the mouths of patients

should be sterilized after use.

The elaboration of these precautions was done to prevent dentist-to-patient transmission of hepatitis B and other blood-and-saliva-born virus infections and also serve as an AIDS-prevention measure. One case has been reported to the CDC where herpes simplex was transmitted by a dental-care worker to more than 20 patients. Also a rise in the numbers of positive tests for hepatitis B has been noted in dentists, suggesting that "current infection-control practices have been insufficient to prevent the transmission of this infectious agent in the dental operatory (5)." Vaccination of dental personnel for hepatitis B is "strongly recommended" by the CDC (5).

Although saliva is not an efficient transmitter of the AIDS virus and no cases have developed to link AIDS-virus transmission to dental practice, there remains an undeniable risk from exposure to blood during dentistry and particularly in oral surgery. There is no reason to suspect that oral-derived blood would be less infectious than blood from other parts of the body.

Following a recommendation that a medical history be obtained from dental patients with particular questions being asked about unintentional weight loss, lymphadenopathy, hepatitis, and current illnesses, the April, 1986, CDC recommendations for dental practice discusses preventative measures (5).

Protective Attire and Barrier Techniques

1. For protection of personnel and patients, gloves must always be worn when touching blood, saliva, or mucous membranes. Gloves must be worn by DHCWs (dental health care workers) when touching blood-soiled items, body fluids, or secretions, as well as surfaces contaminated with them....All work must be completed on one patient, where possible, and the hands must be washed and regloved before performing procedures on another patient. Repeated use of a

single pair of gloves is not recommended, since such use is likely to produce defects in the glove material, which will diminish its value as an effective barrier.

2. Surgical masks and protective eyewear or chin-length plastic face shields must be worn when splashing or spattering of blood or other body fluids is likely, as is common in dentistry.

3. Reusable or disposable gowns, laboratory coats, or uniforms must be worn when clothing is likely to be soiled with blood or other body fluids. If reusable gowns are worn, they may be washed, using a normal laundry cycle. Gowns should be changed at least daily or when visibly soiled with blood.

4. Impervious-backed paper, aluminum foil, or clear plastic wrap may be used to cover surfaces (e.g., light handles or x-ray unit heads) that are difficult or impossible to disinfect that may be contaminated by blood or saliva. The coverings should be removed (while DHCWs are gloved), discarded, and then replaced (after ungloving) with clean material between patients.

5. All procedures and manipulations of potentially infective materials should be performed carefully to minimize the formation of droplets, spatters, and aerosols, where possible. Use of rubber dams, where appropriate, high-speed evacuation, and proper patient positioning should facilitate this process.

Other recommendations contained in the April, 1986, report concern use and care of sharp instruments and needles, sterilization of instruments, cleaning working surfaces, biopsy specimens and disposal of waste materials (5).

Because an AIDS-infected individual may not be aware he has the disease, dentist and hygienist may be the first to recognize some of the symptoms of AIDS in their patients. The presence of oral thrush, the recognition of a recent weight loss, cloudiness or hemorrhages in one or both eyes are symptoms that are sometimes related to

AIDS that might be observed.

The precautions outlined should be followed in the care of all patients to prevent the spread of any infection from patient-to-dentist or dentist-to-patient. Because most seropositive individuals will show no indications of AIDS infection and the increasing prevalence of AIDS in all parts of the United States, preventing the transmission of any infectious agent in a dental setting is one of the most important obligations of dental care. These precautions should be uniformly adopted even among practitioners with a "safe" clientele. Dentistry has entered a new era in regards to infection control.

OPTOMETRISTS

Tears have not been shown to be an efficient transmitter of the AIDS virus, but the virus has been isolated from eye fluids. One method used to inoculate laboratory animals with a virus is to place a quantity of virus in solution and place this solution in the membrane surrounding the eye. Because the effectiveness of this procedure of virus inoculation had been demonstrated on a regular basis the CDC felt in 1982 that it was necessary to recommend precautionary measures to prevent this possible path of virus transmission (1).

No cases of transmission of the AIDS virus exclusively by tears have been documented, but the recommendations given below have not been modified or rescinded.

The following precautions are judged suitable to prevent spread of HTLV-III/LAV and other microbial pathogens that might be present in tears (2). They do not apply to the procedures used by individuals in caring for their own lenses, since the concern is the possible virus transmission between individuals.

1. Health-care professionals performing eye examinations or other procedures involving contact with tears should wash their hands immediately after

a procedure and between patients. Hand washing alone should be sufficient; but when practical and convenient, disposable gloves may be worn The use of gloves is advisable when there are cuts, scratches, or dermatologic lesions on the hands. Use of other protective measures, such as masks, goggles, or gowns, is NOT indicated.

2. Instruments that come into direct contact with external surfaces of the eye should be wiped clean and then disinfected by: (a) a 5-to-10 minute exposure to a fresh solution of 3 % hydrogen peroxide or (b) a fresh solution containing 5,000 parts per million (mg/L) free available chlorine - a 1:10 dilution of common household bleach solution (sodium hypochlorite) or (c) 70% isopropanol. The device should be thoroughly rinsed in tap water and dried before reuse.

3. Contact lenses used in trial fittings should be disinfected between each fitting by one of the following regimens:

a. Disinfection of trial hard lenses with a commercially available hydrogen peroxide contact lens disinfecting solution currently approved for soft contact lenses. (Other hydrogen peroxide preparations may contain preservatives that could discolor the lenses.) Alternatively, most trial hard lenses can be treated with the standard heat disinfection regimen used for soft lenses (70-80 C (172-176 F.) for 10 minutes). Practitioners should check with hard lens suppliers to ascertain which lenses can be safely heat-treated.

b. Rigid gas permeable (RPG) trial fitting lenses can be disinfected using the above hydrogen peroxide disinfection system. RPG lenses may warp if they are heat-disinfected.

c. Soft trial fitting lenses can be disinfected using the same hydrogen peroxide system. Some soft lenses have also been approved for heat disinfection.

Other than hydrogen peroxide, the chemical disinfectants used in standard contact lens solutions have not yet been tested for their activity against HTLV-III/LAV. Until other disinfectant are shown to be suitable, contact lenses used in the eyes of patients suspected or known to be infected with HTLV-III/LAV are most safely handled by hydrogen peroxide disinfection.

As is the case with the dentists mentioned earlier, ophthalmologists may be the first to notice some symptoms of AIDS. Abnormalities in the eyes include retinal hemorrhage caused by cytomegalovirus or periordital Kaposi's sarcoma.

PATHOLOGISTS AND MORTICIANS

1. As part of immediate postmortem care, deceased persons should be identified as belonging to one of these three groups (patients with AIDS; patients with chronic, generalized lymphadenopathy, unexplained weight loss, and/or prolonged fever when the patient's history suggest a risk for AIDS; all hospitalized patients with possible AIDS), and that identification should remain with the body (1).

2. The procedures followed before, during, and after the postmortem examination are similar to those for hepatitis B. All personnel involved in performing an autopsy should wear double gloves, masks, protective eyewear, gowns, waterproof aprons, and waterproof shoe coverings. Instruments and surfaces contaminated during the postmortem examination should be handled as potentially infective items.

3. Morticians should evaluate specific procedures used in providing mortuary care and take appropriate precautions to prevent the parenteral or mucous-membrane exposure of personnel to body fluids.

The recommendations given for the protection of morticians are not very detailed. By assumption, it would appear that the protective measures given under Part 2 in this section would apply. Many morticians are reluctant to provide services for deceased AIDS patients, and some will only provide cremation. The issue of how the body is to be disposed of is one that needs to be addressed by the AIDS patient and his family.

The CDC is presently revising its recommendations, and judging from the present revisions this organization is tending towards more stringent precautions. There is a need for recommendations that will symplify, rather than complicate patient care and to continuously review them in light of recent knowledge about how AIDS is spread.

----

1. Centers for Disease Control, 1982, Acquired immune deficiency syndrome (AIDS); Precautions for clinical and laboratory staffs: Mortality Weekly Report November 5; and, 1983, Acquired immunodeficiency syndrome (AIDS); Precautions for health-care workers and allied professionals: Mortality Weekly Report, September 2; in U.S. public health service recommended precautions for health care workers and allied professionals regarding acquired immunodeficiency syndrome (AIDS),. 1983, U.S. Department of Health & Human Services, U.S. Public Health Service.

2. Centers for Disease Control, 1985, Recommendations for preventing possible transmission of human T-lymphotrophic virus type III/lymphadenopathy-associated virus from tears: Mortality Weekly Report, August 30.

3. Mines, Jonathan, 1985, A 24-month prospective study of the ophthalmologic findings in the acquired immune deficiency syndrome: Poster W-38. International Conference on AIDS, Atlanta, Georgia.

4. Centers for Disease Control, 1986, Recommendations for

preventing transmission of infection with human T-lymphotropic Virus Type III/LAV lymphadenopathy-associated virus during invasive procedures: Mortality Weekly Report, April 11.

5. Centers for Disease Control, 1986, Recommended infection-control practices for dentistry: Weekly Mortality Report, April 18.

POLITICAL AND LEGAL ASPECTS

WHEN REDUCED TO ITS ESSENCE defeating AIDS and caring for those who are infected will cost billions of dollars of which most must come from governmental appropriations. Private groups around the world can and are raising money for psycosocial care, counseling, and dissemination of information about the syndrome; but basic research and the hospital care of increasing numbers of severely ill individuals cannot be effectively financed by private charities.

The costs of treating those with AIDS is anticipated to reach $8 billion in the United States by 1991. The annual budget for publicly-funded research has not been estimated, but appropriations in 1986 alone were $294 million which included $50 million for AIDS research and blood testing by the armed forces. Each hospitalization of an AIDS patient now averages about $14,000. Total treatment costs of an average AIDS patient is presently about $46,000 (1). Although a portion of hospitalization costs are met by private insurance, the high costs of hospitalizations, drugs, and therapies often quickly exhaust insurance benefits as well as consume the private assets of the person being treated.

Most people being treated for the syndrome in the United States are on Medicaid, a government-financed health program, because they no longer have the financial resources to pay for treatment.

Appropriating and designing methods of administering the large amounts of money required to support both research and patient treatment is a political task requiring diligent efforts to insure that the money is effectively used.

In the United States the Centers for Disease Control studies issues dealing with the epidemiology, the growth and methods of spread, of AIDS; the National Institutes of Health considers the basic science of AIDS, the kinds of viruses responsible, their structure, how they grow, and possible biological and chemical methods of defeating them; and the Food and Drug Administration covers the testing of drugs and issues regarding the safety and production of vaccines.

These organizations are overseen by the Department of Health and Human Services whose secretary has a cabinet post position and is directly responsible to the President of the United States. The secretary presents a budget to the President who, in turn, incorporates it into his budget proposal to Congress.

Both Houses of Congress may modify the President's budget, produce an independent budget, or a budget containing features of both. When the budget is passed by both houses, it is sent for approval to the President who must either accept or reject it. He may not at this time use a "line-item veto" to return to Congress one or more parts of the budget for reconsideration while passing the rest.

Members of Congress, particularly those on the health committees of both Houses, have considerable power in determining how much money will be spent each year on AIDS research and to support AIDS patients who are no longer able to pay for their own health care. Working with these committee members as well as with the other members of Congress who may accept, modify, or reject the committee's proposed budget is a vital task which, by default, is mostly being carried by gay AIDS-action organizations.

These organizations, notably the National AIDS Network and affiliated groups, are lobbying Congress and monitoring state legislatures in an attempt to help insure that appropriate, meaningful acts of legislation are passed which take into account protection of the civil rights of those who have AIDS (3).

Why are civil rights important? Putting aside for the moment, but by no means dismissing, the right of every American citizen to equal justice under law, the fact is that gays are, and will remain, the most susceptible and most numerous group infected with the

AIDS virus. If this group is driven underground by repressive legislation, such as threat of quarantine, gays will be more difficult to reach, and/or treat, and any hope of controlling the disease is lost.

Every group working with AIDS has discovered how difficult it is to administer an effective prevention program to IV drug users. Because of possible legal actions, drug users are reluctant to be identified or submit to counseling which could lead to preventing the spread of AIDS and curing their addictions. The must successful approach used thus far has been needle and syringe exchange programs where the person presenting injection equipment for exchange is not identified.

CONFIDENTIALITY OF TEST RESULTS

The largest group that have been universally tested for AIDS antibodies have been members of the United States Army and prospective recruits. This approach has opened the way for private companies to use the test for screening of potential, and present, employees. Some states, such as California, have made it illegal to force someone to take the test. While such legislation may prevent some abuse of the test, what about the case where an employer might require a person to take the test as a condition of employment or in order to be eligible for health insurance (4)?

Unless legally prevented, a candidate for a job might be required to sign a waver of his rights to refuse the test and of his rights of confidentiality. The bottom line so far as an employer might be, "If you don't take this test, we will not consider your job application."

Universal testing is of doubtful usefulness. Even if a person tested negatively for the virus on one test, a week, or a month, or a year later he may give a positive test as a result of a more recent sexual contact. Only in a closed institution, such as a prison, might universal testing be of potential use if seropositive individuals were segregated from the rest of the population. This approach would generate its problems.

If a person's name is linked with the results of testing at any stage in the testing process, there is a risk that the test results could be disclosed. The approach used by most anonymous testing centers is to use either a fictitious name or a number to identify the person, releasing the test result only to him on presentation of a matching document, and then destroying the documents.

The only thing retained by the testing center would be the number of people tested; their age, race, sex, and symptoms; and the test results.

In the case of a doctor treating a patient that the physician has reason to believe may have symptoms of an AIDS-related illness, assurances of preserving the confidentiality of the test results is a serious consideration. The safest presently available method would be for the patient to go to an anonymous testing site, have his blood tested, and then give the results to his physician. If this is impractical, then the physician should develop a mode of operation where he can draw the blood and send it to such a center for testing or develop another method to insure that confidentiality will be maintained.

Some state legislatures, such as in South Carolina and Colorado, have considered legislation that would require a physician to report the names and addresses of any person diagnosed with AIDS to the state health officer. The danger of this approach is that the confidentiality of this information will not be guaranteed, and the names might be "leaked" to other state agencies or authorities (4).

The concept of reporting the names of AIDS or ARC cases or identifying seropositive persons to state health officers is of little use. If the purpose is to gather statistical data, this information is already available on a state-wide basis from the CDC. If data compilation is the purpose of the reporting procedure, then why is identification of the individual needed?

If such measures are taken under the cry of "protecting the public safety," then some other measures must be necessary to implement this "protective" activity. Proposals have included unforceable prohibitions such as making it illegal for seropositive individuals to engage in sex, mandatory testing for those who are considered "at risk" for AIDS, and the quarantine or chemical castration of seropositive individuals who "knowingly engage in hazardous sexual activity."

Such measures have appeared in bills introduced in several state legislatures in the United States during 1985-56. Such proposals serve to make gays suspicious of the motives of governmental agencies, resist voluntary testing, and less likely to seek medical treatment for fear of discrimination (3).

The matter of quarantine, or in practical terms, jailing of infected individuals, was forcefully brought to the public's attention from the widely-publicized case of a male prostitute in Houston, who announced that even though he had AIDS, he would continue "to ply his trade" despite a court order that he desist. Under such circumstances, and only after all other measures have failed and hearings held to protect the civil rights of the individual, does quarantine make any sense. Quarantine should be considered as a last resort, and state health officers already have the power to order the quarantine of a person whose infectivity status and activities make him a deadly threat to the public (4).

Prisons in the United States reported 766 cases of AIDS from a total of 84 federal, state, county, and city institutions according to a March 28, 1986, report of the CDC. This study documented a variety of solutions used by these institutions to prevent the spread of AIDS. Nine of the institutions had no policy, two had no segregation of infected inmates, six segregated only AIDS cases, 13 segregated AIDS and ARC cases, and 21 segregated AIDS, ARC, and seropositive individuals. No cases of AIDS had been reported in correctional staffs. The report concluded, "The apparent lack of reported AIDS cases among correctional staff as a result from casual contact is consistent with previous findings that the risk of HTLV-III/LAV transmission in occupational settings is extremely low...(5)."

This report also stated that IV drug use was the primary factor in AIDS infection in inmates and pointed out that the highest rate of AIDS cases among inmates occurred in institutions in New York and New Jersey where IV drug users formed a larger part of the prisons' populations than elsewhere in the United States (5).

Two issues facing correctional institutions are testing of inmates and preventing the transmission of AIDS. In speaking of testing, the CDC made no recommendations, but pointed out that, "testing could, however, pose difficulties for a number of correctional facilities. In some jurisdictions, legal and policy provisions may currently prohibit testing. Many correctional systems assert that, if testing is done, the results cannot be kept confidential (and) seropositive inmates could face a range of problems, including the possibility of physical harm (5)."

It would appear that unless provisions are available for transfer of all seropositive individuals to a separate prison or to another part of an existing facility that inmate testing, by itself, would be of little use.

Few correctional officers will openly that sexual activity takes place in their institutions. Since these activities "do not exist," steps like distribution of condoms or selling them in a prison cannot be promoted. Education is the only approach available to many correctional officers to prevent transmission of AIDS. If condoms were included in a packet of AIDS-educational materials, this might be a more "politically acceptable" method of providing condoms to inmates. Many gay organizations now distribute condoms enclosed in match-book covers printed with "safer sex" guidelines.

After the first distribution of condoms, it is likely that a "black market" trade in them would evolve within the prison that would result in the condoms reaching the more sexually active members of the prison population. Once it is generally perceived within the prison that the condoms have value, the chances of their being wasted are reduced.

LEGAL ISSUES

A large number of legal questions have been raised in the United States in regard to AIDS. Some of these issues involve society's obligations to protect an institutionalized individual. While other cases were taken to court by people who were unknowingly infected (or exposed) by a person who knew he had AIDS or by a blood transfusion as well as another group of cases hinging on violations of civil rights or discrimination.

Many of these cases are in the process of making their way through the nation's courts and a body of case law about AIDS is slowly evolving. The general trend of court decisions are (4):

1. Activities of correctional officers to test, or choose not to test, inmates have been upheld.

2. The rights of blood banks to keep the identity of blood donors confidential have been upheld.

3. Children with AIDS or seropositive children have been allowed to continue school.

4. In the absence of a demonstrated "clear and present danger" to the community, individuals with AIDS and those who are seropositive retained their rights to jobs, health services, and equal housing.

The liability of an individual who knows he has AIDS or is seropositive and infects, or exposes to infection, another party is now being decided in several cases.

Perhaps the case that has most attracted the public's attention is a suit filed against the estate of Rock Hudson by a person claiming to be a sex partner. The latter, even though he did not contract the AIDS virus, is claiming damages for "pain and suffering" on grounds that Hudson had AIDS at the time of the encounter, but did not tell him. This case is still before the courts.

Using an an analogy cases that have been decided in favor of those infected with herpes by a person who knew that he carried the disease, suits have been filed against sex partners for supposedly infecting others with the AIDS virus. Because of the long incubation period of AIDS, such suits are difficult to prove as there is no presently known method of identifying a particular person as the transmitter of the virus.

A plaintiff can claim that the virus was transmitted by a defendant, but unless the plaintiff can prove to a jury that the virus came from the defendant, and no other possible source, the case is open to question. The identification of a single sexual partner other than the defendant during the previous eight years, unless that partner could be located, agree to be tested, and proved to be seronegative, would probably cloud the case to such a degree that no clear finding of fact could be made. The fact that the defendant might refuse to have his blood tested could not be used as evidence.

If a defendant had progressed to ARC or AIDS and there was convincing evidence that he had been the plaintiff's only sex partner during the previous eight years, a sufficiently strong case might be presented that would result in a jury award for damages.

----

1. Curran, James W., 1986, The epidemiology of AIDS; current status and future prospects: Centers for Disease Control, Atlanta, Georgia U.S.A., Second International Conference on AIDS, Paris, France.
2. MacDonald, Gary, 1986, Update and discussion on AIDS-related issues; political, civil rights, services, legal and people with AIDS: Seventh National Lesbian/Gay Health Conference, Washington, D.C.
3. Levi, Jeff, 1986, Update and discussion on AIDS-related issues; political, civil rights, services, legal and people with AIDS: Seventh National Lesbian/Gay Health Conference, Washington, D.C.
4. Centers for Disease Control, 1986, Acquired immunodeficiency syndrome in correctional facilities; a report of the National Institute of Justice and the American Correctional Association: Weekly Mortality Report, March 28.

GLOSSARY

Acyclovir An antiviral drug effective against herpes simplex. A similar drug, DHPG (Burroughs Wellcome BWB759U), has been used for experimental treatment of infections caused by cytomegalovirus, another of the herpesviruses.

Adenopathy Swelling of the lymph nodes due to disease.

Adenovirus (AV) One of a large number of similar viruses often found in the stool, urine, lymph nodes, nerves, muscles tissue, and digestive tracts of AIDS patients which may cause upper respiratory infections.

Aerosol A method of drug delivery where a drug is aspirated through the breathing passages into the lungs to help avoid toxic effects to the kidney, liver, and spleen. This therapy is now being used to administer pentamidine to AIDS patients at the Memorial Sloan-Kettering Cancer Center in New York and the San Francisco Medical Center.

Agar A culture media made from an extract of red alga often used as a host material for growing bacteria.

AIDS (Acquired Immunodeficiency Syndrome) A group of diseases, a syndrome, caused by the HTLV-III (LAV) human retrovirus which is destructive to the body's immune system, leaving it open to a variety of diseases including uncommon types of cancer and pneumonias.

AIDS-related complex (ARC) 1. A group of symptoms which appear to be related to an infection of the AIDS virus. 2. A group of characteristic opportunistic infections to which AIDS patients are disposed, and the symptoms caused by these infections.

Alopeica   The loss of hair, which frequently occurs   in patients   undergoing chemotherapy for cancer and in other diseases such as AIDS where cell-killing,   or   cytotoxic, drugs are used.

Alpha-2 recombinant interferon   Used in   France   by   R. Rozenbaum   as an agent against KS.   This author reported that patients responded favorably to this treatment.

Ameboasos   Infestation of the body   with   one-celled animals called amebas,   particularly   Emtamoeba   hystolytica which   may cause amebic dysentery, colon ulcers, or liver diseases.

Amphetamines   An often addictive central nervous   system stimulant   used   in pill form as an   "upper"   to   produce extreme energy and unusual excitement.   Investigated as a cofactor   in   causing the onset of serious   complications resulting from infection with the AIDS virus.   No   positive link has been established,   but the recreational use of   amphetamines   or any drugs among high risk groups   is not recommended.

Amyl nitrite (amyl)   An organic liquid   compound   ingested   by sniffing,   which is reputed to heighten sexual passions.   Commonly used by the gay population and often considered   as a possible cofactor in the contraction   of AIDS.   No firm evidence has positively linked the use of amyl nitrite with AIDS,   although linkage with the development of Kaposi's sarcoma is suggested by several   studies.

Anal intercourse   Penetration of the anus by the penis of the dominant partner.

Anemia   A reduction of the number of red blood cells   in the blood which reduces its oxygen-carrying capacity.

Anergy 1. The loss or weakening of the body's immunity to an irritating agent, or antigen. The strength of the body's immune response is often quantitatively measured by means of a skin test where a solution containing an antigen is injected immediately under the skin. 2. A lack of energy or becoming tired after slight exertions.

Anorexia A loss of interest in food or eating caused by a lack of appetite. This condition may be caused by disease, depression, or drug addiction.

Ansamycin (LM 427) A drug which in test cultures inhibits the growth and reproduction of <u>Mycobacterium</u> <u>avium</u>, a cause of a type of tuberculosis which is a common opportunistic infection in AIDS patients. In limited human trials 30 percent of the patients improved and the drug appeared to be well tolerated, but its effectiveness remains to be demonstrated.

Antibody A globulin protein produced in response to a specific infectious agent which may neutralize toxins and antigens, cause bacteria or foreign cells to stick together, or cause antigens to precipitate from solutions. Produced by plasma cells in the lymphatic system.

Antibiotic Any of a group of drugs, usually derived from living organisms, that are used to combat bacterial infections. Common examples of such drugs are penicillin and streptomycin.

Antigen A substance, usually a protein or a carbohydrate, that causes protective antibodies to be produced by the organism that has been invaded by the antigen.

Antimoniotungstate (HPA 23) A drug used in trials as a possible treatment for patients with Kaposi's sarcoma. This drug is also used as an antiviral drug to inhibit the reproduction of viruses by not allowing the reverse transcriptase activity of the viruses to function. This drug is also thought to activate the body's killer T-cells. In limited human trials, the drug inhibited the spread of the HTLV-III virus, but the virus resumed activity when the drug was discontinued. This drug is suggested as being potentially useful as a part of an immune restoration treatment.

Antimortem Prior to death.

Antimycotic A drug that inhibits the growth and/or reproduction of fungi.

Antimycobacterial A drug or treatment that kills or discourages the growth of mycobacterial infections such as Mycobacterium avium and Mycobacterium tuberculosis, both of which may occur as opportunistic infections in AIDS patients

ARC (AIDS-related complex) Symptoms which appear to be related to infection by the AIDS virus. They include an unexplained, chronic deficiency of white blood cells (leukopenia) or a poorly functioning lymphatic system with swelling of the lymph nodes (lymphadenopathy) lasting for more than three months without the opportunistic infections require for a diagnosis of AIDS.

ARV (AIDS-related (or associated) retrovirus) A retrovirus which is thought to be responsible for or associated with AIDS. The virus which causes AIDS has been identified as the HTLV-III retrovirus, also known as LAV, and in 1986 was renamed HIV, replacing the names previously given the AIDS virus.

Assay Either a qualitative or a quantitative test, such as the qualitative ELISA or Western blot test for AIDS, to determine the presence and/or amount of any given factor, agent, or substance being sought in an analysis.

Asymptomatic Without symptoms. Usually used in AIDS literature to describe a person who has a positive reaction to one of several tests for AIDS antibodies, but who shows no external symptoms of the disease.

Autoantibody An antibody that is active against some of the tissues of the organism that produced it.

Autoantigen An antigen that stimulates the production of antibodies which attack the body's own tissues, as occurs in autoimmune diseases.

Autoimmune disease A disease in which the body's own immune system attacks some organ or other tissues within the body.

Azotemia Presence of urea or other nitrogen compounds in the blood. This is usually caused by partial or complete kidney failure.

AZT (azidothymidine) A drug developed by Burroughs Wellcome for use against PCP and approved for wide-spread testing in 1986. This drug has serious side effects including suppression of bone marrow function, resulting in a severe anemia that may require blood transfusions to correct.

B-lymphocytes A type of cell produced by the body's lymphatic system to combat infections and diseases. In AIDS patients the functional ability of both the B and the T-lymphocytes is damaged, with the T-lymphocytes being the principal site of infection by the AIDS virus.

Bacteremia A disease caused by bacterial infection, particularly bacterial infections in the bloodstream.

Bactrim An antibiotic consisting of the drugs sulfamethoxazole and trimethoprim that limited human trials demonstrated to be successful for preventing reoccurrences of <u>Pneumocystis</u> <u>carinii</u> pneumonia after successful treatment of the disease with other drugs.

Baseline Information gathered at the beginning of a study from which variations found in the study are measured. Sometimes referred to as "a datum" or "base datum."

Biopsy The extraction and examination of a piece of tissue to determine if infectious or cancerous diseases are present.

Biopsychosocial A unified approach to the treatment of diseases where the needs of the body, the mind, and the ability of the patient to function in society are considered.

Bisexual An individual who is sexually attracted to members of both sexes.

Blastogenesis Reproduction of cells, viruses, bacteria, fungi, and plants by budding, rather than by sexual reproduction.

Bleomycin sulfate A drug found by J.P. Clauvel of Saint Louis Hospital in Paris to have moderate activity against KS with 50 percent of patients exhibiting improvement.

Bone marrow transplant A technique in which bone marrow from one person is injected into another person's bones in order to reconstitute the body's immune system. Among AIDS patients bone marrow transplants have been restricted to identical twins. Without a simultaneous drug therapy, transplants among AIDS patients have resulted in only temporarily restoring the body's immune system before also failing under the attack of the AIDS virus.

Bronchoscopy Visual examinations of the bronchial passages of the lungs through a tube of an endoscope inserted into the upper lungs or extraction of material from the lungs by means of a bronchoscope.

Burkitt-like lymphoma A lymphatic cancer which involves not only the lymphatic and the associated reticuloendothelial system, but also other body tissues. This disease is most common in Central Africa. It is thought to be possibly caused by the Epstein-Barr virus.

BWB759U (9-(2-hydrox-1-(hydroxymethyl) ethoxymethyl) **guanine** Gary N. Holland at the UCLA School of Medicine in Los Angeles found that 16 or 18 patients treated with this drug responded favorably with partial or total remission of progressive retinopathy caused by cytomegalovirus infection.

Candida esophagitis An infection of the esophagus caused by the fungus Candida. One of this family of fungi, Candida albicans, is responsible for thrush infections of the mouth.

Candidiasis Infection by any of the Candida fungi which may be localized in the mouth, esophagus or skin, but which may also infect the bloodstream.

CDC (Centers for Disease Control) The Centers for Disease Control are located in Atlanta, Georgia, with a sister organization called the National Institutes of Health in Bethesda, Maryland. The CDC is under the direction of the Alcohol, Drug Abuse, and Mental Health Administration of the Public Health Service of the U.S. Department of Health and Human Services.

Central nervous system (CNS) The brain, spinal cord and associated tissues such as the myelin sheaths which surround them.

Chemotherapy The treatment, mostly of cancer, by the use of a series of cytotoxic drugs which attack cancerous cells. This treatment commonly has adverse side effects which may include the temporary loss of the body's natural immunity to infections, loss of hair, digestive upset, and a general feeling of illness. Although unpleasant, the adverse effects of treatment are tolerated considering the life-threatening nature of cancers usually treated by chemotherapy.

Clindamycin A drug used with limited success against cryptosporidiosis when administered with quinine.

Clone A genetically identical replication of a living cell which is valuable for the investigation and reproduction of test cultures.

Cocaine A white, addictive alkaloid that has medicinal uses as a pain-relieving drug, but cocaine and a derivative called crack are now commonly used as an illegal recreational drug taken through the nostrils, injection into veins with heroin (speedballing), or smoked. Although a causative connection has not been established between cocaine use and AIDS, the use of this drug weakens a person's resolve not to engage in unsafe sexual practices. Frequent users of this drug may develop cocainism, a morbidly depressed state which contributes to psychological problems resulting from AIDS.

Cofactor An agent or perhaps a combination of agents that may cause an attack of AIDS to begin after a latent period of up to five years or predispose the person to infection by the virus.

Colonoscopy Direct visual examination of the colon (lower intestine) by means of a flexible instrument with fiberoptic filaments, an endoscope, which allows the interior of the intestine to be illuminated for visual examination or photography.

Cotrimoxazole A drug used in initial therapy for treatment of _Pneumocystis carinii_ pneumonia.

Cohort A group of any size which has been designated for study.

Coronavirus One of the concanavalin viruses.

Cotrimoxarole A drug used for treatment and to prevent reoccurrence of PCP.

Cryptococcal meningitis Infection by a cryptococcus fungus causing an inflammation of one or more of the meninges membranes surrounding the brain and spinal cord. Meningitis may also be caused by viral or bacterial infections.

Cryptococcus neoformans (Sp.) A species of cryptococcus fungus that may infect the lungs causing a flu-like disease. It may also spread through the bloodstream and infect other organs, such as the brain. The cryptococcus fungi is common in chicken and pigeon droppings. The disease is spread by breathing airborne spores. Crypto-coccus neoformans has been observed to be poorly encapsulated when associated with AIDS.

Cryptosporidia A protozoan parasite, Cryptosporidium, that may infect either the intestinal or respiratory tract of reptiles, birds, and mammals. Before the outbreak of AIDS in 1981 only seven cases had been reported in humans. The organism causes a severe, unrelenting diarrhea in AIDS patients, but only mild symptoms in the healthy. An ELISA test is available for determining if antibodies to this parasite are present in the blood.

Cryptosporidiosis The disease caused by the parasite, Cryptosporidium, which may be localized in either the intestinal or respiratory tract.

Crytotoxic To be killed by cold temperatures.

CS-85 A drug under development at Emory University in Atlanta which appears to work similarly to AZT against PCP infections, but which is claimed by Raymond F. Schinazi to be from 10 to 100 times less toxic from the results of in-vitro trials.

Cytomegalovirus One of a group of herpesviruses which can cause retinitis of the eyes, pneumonia, and infection of nervous system and/or intestinal tract. In AIDS patients it often causes long-lasting severe diarrhea that has proved to be difficult to treat with existing drugs. This virus is sometimes also accompanied by a simultaneous infection with <u>Shigella</u> <u>flexneri</u> bacteria.

Cytotoxic drugs Drugs primarily used to treat cancers which are also deadly to rapidly-multiplying healthy cells. These drugs often have injurious side affects when they attack healthy cells.

Cytotoxic (killer) T-cells These cells produced by the body's lymphatic system secrete a poison when activated by having a foreign substance presented to the T-cell by a macrophage. These cells are found in the blood and circulate through the body.

D-penicillamine A drug ordinarily given to people with arthritis which according to Richard Schulof of George Washington University appeared in first human trials to keep the AIDS virus from reproducing, but which has the undesireable effect of supressing production of T-cells.

Dementia An irrecoverable mental disorder resulting in the loss of the ability to reason and logically plan activities. The AIDS virus either acting alone or in conjunction with <u>Toxoplasma</u> <u>gondii,</u> a protozoan parasite, and/or other infections causes damage in the form of lesions in the brain or disseminated infestations of the brain and spinal cord. Such brain damage is the organic cause of the dementia observed in late-stage AIDS. Dementia is not always present, but is common. Remissions have been observed, but these are usually only temporary interruptions of the steady progression of disease.

Detoxification 1. The neutralization or removal of toxic substances from the blood. 2. Also applied to drug and alcohol treatment processes where the patient's use of the abused substance is reduced in stages to the point of nonuse, and the body is allowed to eliminate the toxic materials.

DFMO (eflornithine hydrochloride) An ornithine deriva- tive drug used for treatment of PCP or cryptococcosis that was found by J.L.R. Barlow to be effective in con- trolling the PCP parasite in 26 of 27 patients.

DHPG (9 (1,3 dihydroxpropoxymethyl) guanine) Found by A.S. Tyms of St. Mary's Hospital Medical School in London to be a potent inhibitor of CMV in vitro and in limited clinical trials.

DHCW Dental health care worker.

Diaminodiphenylsulfone (dapsone) A drug successfully used for treatment of Pneumocystis carinii pneumonia in rats, but which was found to have adverse side effects in limited human testing. This drug has been successfully used for treatment of leprosy and bacterial infections.

Diarrhea Uncontrolled, loose, and frequent bowel move- ments. In AIDS patients periods of diarrhea may last for months or years with up to 20 bowel movements per day. Diarrhea is a factor in the rapid weight loss frequently observed in AIDS patients. It may be caused by protozoan or bacterial infection, or both types of infections may be present at the same time.

Dihydromycoplanecin-A A drug exhibiting in vitro activity against Mycobacterium avium pheumonia.

DNA The molecular chain, deoxyribonucleic acid, found in genes within the nucleus of each cell, which carries the genetic information that enables cells to reproduce.

Dysphoria A general feeling of illness and discontent without apparent cause.

Electrophorentically purified (or identified) A method of determining the composition of cell proteins by the speed and direction of their movement through a gel in response to an electrical charge.

ELISA (enzyme-linked immunosorbent assay) A test which
determines if antibodies to a given agent are present in
blood samples. The ELISA test for AIDS has a high detection rate, but may give a few (1-3 percent) false-positive results on the first administration of the test. A
negative result on the test means that there are no AIDS
antibodies present in the sample being tested. The lack
of antibodies may mean that the system has not had a
chance to develop antibodies because of a recent exposure
or, in advanced cases of AIDS, that the antibody producing mechanisms of the lymph system have been destroyed.
Because of this, only positive test results are considered to be meaningful. Another ELISA test is available for the detection of cryptosporidia, a protozoan
parasite, that may infect the respiratory or intestinal
tracts of AIDS patients.

Encephalitis Inflammation of the brain cells caused by a
virus infection. Among the viruses linked with this
disease are those which cause herpes simplex and mumps.
The disease may be mild, but it may be life threatening
to those having impaired immune systems, such as AIDS
patients.

Endemic area An area where a disease or a disease-pro-
ducing organism originated or is customarily found.

Endoscopy A direct visual examination of one of the
body's cavities, such as the lungs or colon (lower intestine), by means of an endoscope with fiberoptic filaments, which allows the interior of the intestine to be
illuminated for visual examination or photography.

Endonuclease protein A protein derived from within the
nucleus of a virus.

ENV A virus gene that determines the properties of the
viral envelope.

Epidemiologic Pertaining to the study of epidemic

diseases, particularly in regard to the spread of such diseases.

Epstein-Barr virus A herpes-like virus which has been found in people with Burkitt's lymphoma and infectious mononucleosis.

Esophageal Having to do with the esophagus as in esophageal infections.

Esophagitis Inflammation of the esophagus.

Ethambutol An antibacterial agent used in the treatment of mycobacterial tuberculosis, but which does not appear to be active against other bacteria, fungi, or viruses.

Ethionamide Used with other drugs in the treatment of tuberculosis and, in particular, against mycobacterial tuberculosis.

Etiologic agent The causative agent of an infection, condition or disease.

Factor VIII The clotting agent in the blood. This material is frequently concentrated from blood products and administered to hemophiliacs whose blood lacks this clotting agent.

Fansidar A drug sometimes given as a protection against a relapse of a person successfully treated for Pneumocystis carinii pheumonia.

Failure to thrive A disease of infants where, for whatever reason, they fail to grow or react in a normal manner.

Febrile episodes Periods of relatively elevated body temperatures in a patient.

FELV (feline leukemia virus) A virus for which an inactivated whole virus vaccine has been developed to control this disease in cats.

Fibroblast cells Cells which circulate in the blood and aid in blood clotting.

Filaria A nematode found in the blood and intestines of man and other mammals which may infect the lymphatic system. Filaria is usually transmitted by a mosquito bite.

Fisting Insertion of the fist into the rectum of the submissive sexual partner by the dominant sexual partner.

Flucytosine A drug used to combat <u>Cryptococcus</u> <u>neoformans</u> infections, but treatment with this drug or with amphotericine B has been effective in about 40 percent of the patients on which this therapy has been tried.

Foscarnet (trisodium phosphonoformate) A drug used at the Calud Bernard hospital in France for treating cytomegalovirus infections.

Frank AIDS A case of infection with the HTLV-III virus with one or more opportunistic infections that fulfills the Centers for Disease Control's definition of AIDS.

Fungicide A chemical that kills fungus infections and destroys the reproductive spores of the fungus.

Gag This gene provides coding for the group antigen of the AIDS virus.

Gallium imaging This technique provides for early PCP detection and is particularly useful for discovering or determining the results of treatment for multifocal, extrapulmonary disease.

Gamma globulin A fraction of the blood that contains antibodies. This may be given to a person whose immune system has failed.

Gamma interferon A T-cell-derived stimulating substance which suppresses virus reproduction, stimulates other T-cells, and activates macrophage cells. Although this substance appeared to be initially attractive in laboratory cultures, it has not proved to be effective when administered to AIDS patients in limited human testing.

Ganciclovir A drug used by Gary N. Holland of the University of California at Los Angeles as an agent to help fight eye disease caused by cytomegalovirus. At present, the drug is administered on a continual basis by IV injection.

Genomes The combined set of chromosomes providing the genetic blueprint for reproducing the AIDS virus.

Giant cells Cells of unusually large size with several nuclei found in the bone marrow, spleen, and healing tissues in healthy individuals but which are also found as cancerous cells in the central nervous system and in lymph nodes in many AIDS cases.

Global distress A general psychological distress with multiple symptoms.

Global question A question that seeks a general response and covers many aspects of a particular subject that might later be examined by more specific questions.

Glycoprotein The envelope protein of a virus.

Gonorrhea A sexually transmitted venereal disease caused by Neisseria gonorrhoeae which may localize in the sex organs, the mouth, or in the anal cavity of the infected person. Presently being considered as a possible cofactor that may cause a dormant AIDS infection to become active or predispose a person to an AIDS infection.

Granulocyte-macrophage progenitor cell A granular leukocyte cell in the bone marrow of variable form that changes into macrophage cells which enter the blood stream and combats infection by engulfing foreign bodies.

Granulocyte A granular white blood cell or leukocyte.

Granuloma A granular tumor which is most often developed in the lymphatic system.

Green monkeys (Cercopithecus Sp.) A monkey, native to central Africa in which an AIDS-like virus (simian AIDS virus) has been found.

Haitian A native of Haiti, a country which shares the Caribbean island of Hispaniola with the Dominican Republic.

HCW Health care worker.

Helper-inducer T-cells A type of white blood cell, called a lymphocyte or a T-4 cell, which is produced by the lymph glands. In AIDS it is the T-4 cells that become cancerous after being infected by the HTLV-III virus.

Hematology The study of the blood.

Hematologic Relating to blood or the study of blood.

Hemophiliac A person whose blood will not easily clot. People having this inherited blood disease are commonly known as "bleeders."

Hemophilus influenzae (Sp.) A bacteria which is the cause of meningitis and some respiratory infections.

Hepatitis A disease of the liver which may be caused by viral agents introduced into the body by blood products, shared needles, sexual activity, or contact with the body waste products of an infected individual. Three forms of hepatitis are recognized: hepatitis A, hepatitis B, and non-A, non-B hepatitis. Hepatitis B is generally the most serious of the three types.

Hepatomegaly Enlargement of the liver.

Heroin An addictive crystalline derivative of morphine injected into the bloodstream by drug abusers. Injection of drugs, and particularly sharing needles between drug users, have been demonstrated to account for much of the spread of AIDS among heroin users.

Herpes simplex This virus, Herpesvirus hominis, is responsible for blisters and inflammations of the pubic area and sex organs of men and women. It is primarily transmitted by sexual activities including mouth or hand-genital contact during sex. In patients with AIDS or others whose immune system are not functioning adequately, herpes simplex can spread into the bloodstream and infect other organs and cause encephalitis in the brain. A newborn can be infected by herpes during birth and, because its immune system is not fully developed, suffer serious damage to his internal organs.

Herpes zoster This herpes virus is responsible for chicken pox in children and shingles in adults. Herpes zoster in an AIDS patient can cause intense nerve pain, blistering of the skin above the site of the pain, possible loss of feeling in the face, and infection of the eyes which may result in blindness.

Herpesvirus Any of the herpes viruses.

Histopathologic The examination of diseased tissues.

Histoplasmosis A fungus infection, commonly of the lungs, caused by the fungus <u>Histoplasma</u> <u>capsulatum</u>. This fungus is commonly found in bird and/or bat droppings in the Ohio and Mississippi Valley region, the Caribbean Islands and in parts of the Northeast U.S. It is spread by breathing in the spores of the fungus. The most definitive test for the fungus has been from fungal stains and bone marrow cultures. Blood testing has proved to be less reliable.

HIV (human immunodeficiency virus) A name proposed in 1986 to be used for the AIDS virus to replace HTLV-III, LAV, and ARV previously used to designate the virus.

Homophobia A fear of homosexuals.

Homosexual One whose sexual preference is for persons of the same sex.

Horizontal transmission The transmission of AIDS to other members of a household or work place without sexual contact. This term like "casual contact" is a general term. No studies as of 1986 have demonstrated that horizontal transmission of AIDS occurs in normal family life, although one case was reported where a mother became infected by performing home care for a severely ill child who had AIDS. In this case the mother was frequently exposed to the child's blood and is presumed to have contracted the virus through this unusual and repeated exposure.

HPA 23 (ammonium 21-tungsto-9-antimoniate) An antiviral drug on experimental trial at the Pasteur Institute in France that inhibits reverse transcriptase activity in the AIDS virus.

HTLV-I (Human T-4 Cell Lymphothropic Virus, Type I; also sometimes known as Human T-4 Cell Leukemia Virus I) One of three types of viruses known to be associated with leukemia, a disease in which the body's natural ability to produce white blood cells to combat infectious agents has failed. This virus is thought to have originated in Africa in the 16th Century.

HTLV-II (Human T-4 Cell Lymphotrophic Virus, Type II; also sometimes known as Human T-4 Cell Leukemia Virus II) The second known variety of virus known to be associated with leukemia.

HTLV-III (Human T-4 Cell Lymphotrophic Virus, Type III; also known as LAV and sometimes referred to as a Human T-4 Cell Leukemia Virus III) This is the virus that is the causative agent for AIDS. It infects the lymphatic system and causes a cancer which reduces the ability of the system to produce lymphocytes and, as a consequence, to fight infectious diseases. This virus is also thought to be of African origin.

HTLV-IV (Human T-4 Cell Lymphotrophic Virus, Type IV) A new virus identified at the National Cancer Institute in 1986 from blood derived from West Africans. The possible pathologic effects of this virus are now under investigation.

Hybridomas The combination of a human plasma cell with a myeloma (cancer cell) so that the cancer produces a large number of antibodies in test animals which may be purified and injected into human patients.

Hypergammaglobulinemia A near absence of the gamma globulin component of the blood which contains antibodies.

Hypergammaglobulinemic A person who suffers from hypergammaglobulinemia.

Hypertension High blood pressure.

Hypotension Low blood pressure.

Hypoglycemia Low blood sugar level.

Hypoxia Starvation of the tissues in the body because of a lack of oxygen either being absorbed through the lungs or transmitted by the blood, as is the case with people having advanced anemia.

ICRF-159 A drug used in non-AIDS related cases of Kaposi's sarcoma in Africa with success, but unsuccessful in trials of AIDS-related Kaposi's sarcoma in the U.S.

Immune modulators Any of several drugs which attempt to enhance or control the functions of the body's immune system.

Immunodeficiency disease A disease where the body loses its ability to fight infections through a failure of the body's immune system.

Immunoflourescence A type of test where groups of stained cells or antibodies are examined under fluorescent light at high magnifications. This test is sensitive for detection of AIDS if the virus occurs in the cells being examined.

Immunoglobulin (Ig_) Any of five types of immunoglobulins which are capable of acting as antibodies.

Immunological Relating to the body's immune system.

Immunomodulator Any substance or drug which controls the activity of the immune system.

Immunopathogenic An infection, substance, or drug that destroys or damages the body's immune system.

Immunosorbent A form of testing whereby the antibodies produced by the body to fight an infecting agent are absorbed onto an agent where they can be detected by color change, electric response, or other methods.

IMREG 1 A drug which accelerates the production of a patient's T-4 cells. Initial clinical trials have been successful in increasing a patient's ability to resist infection and to restore immune function. Trials with this drug are continuing.

Imuthiol (diethyldithiocarbonate) A study reported by W.

Brewton of the Institute Merieux in Lyon, France, indicated that this drug had a possible use as an immunores-
torative agent in the treatment of AIDS.

Infarcts The interruption of the flow of blood to a
group of tissue because of rupture or constriction of the
blood vessel. Sometimes found in AIDS patients with eye
diseases.

Infection The introduction of a foreign agent into the
body that is capable of destroying the host tissue and
reproducing itself.

Infusion The introduction of fluid into the body or a
group of tissues commonly through an intravenous (IV)
drip.

Interferon alpha A A protein produced by cells exposed
to a virus that has been shown to inhibit the growth of
HTLV-III in cell culture testing. Interferon has the
property of protecting unexposed cells from the virus
that generated its production.

Intramuscular injection (IM) Injection into the muscle
tissue of the body rather than being infused into the
bloodstream or taken through the mouth.

Interleukin-2 A growth factor that stimulates the production of T-cells.

Intravenous (IV) Introduced into the vein, as by using a
drip.

Isopronisine A synthetic lymphokine which is designed to
induce more rapid reproduction of T-4 cells.

Isospora belli (Sp.) A protozoan often found in the
small intestine of man that usually causes no pathologic symptoms. In persons with AIDS this parasites may
reproduce very rapidly and cause Isosporiasis.

Klevsiella pneumonia (Sp.) A species of bacteria that can cause pneumonia and was once believed to be the exclusive cause of the disease.

Kaposi's sarcoma (KS) A previously uncommon form of cancer which attacks the connective tissue, bones, cartilage, and muscles of the body. The cancer may spread and also attack the eyes. If the cancerous area is near the surface of the skin, boils inches in length may develop. This disease was almost completely restricted to elderly men and to natives of Central Africa. Experimental work has shown that the AIDS-related Kaposi's sarcoma and the Central African variety respond differently to some types of medications. In the absence of other opportunistic infections Kaposi's sarcoma responds to long-term vinblastine therapy.

LAS (lymphadenopathy syndrome) A disease of the lymphatic system which results in the failure to produce lymphocytes, a white blood cell necessary for the protection of the body against infections. The syndrome may be caused by infection of the lymph with the AIDS virus, HTLV-III, which causes a lymphoma or cancer of the lymph system.

LAV (Lymphadenopathy Associated Virus) Another name for the AIDS virus, more commonly known in the United States as HTLV-III. Those who engage in the study of the protein composition of viruses maintain that there are differences between the French-identified LAV and the American-identified HTLV-III viruses, but the symptoms and results of infection by these viruses are apparently identical.

LAV 2 (Lymphadenopathy Associated Virus Type 2) This virus was identified in 1986 from blood drawn from a West African man. This virus may be the same as HTLV-IV. The pathologic effects of either of these viruses have not been established, but some workers suggest that it is benign in man. Both of these viruses have closer similarities to the simian AIDS virus than does HTLV-III/LAV (HIV), and some workers consider HTLV-IV/LAV 2 to be a possible parent of the AIDS virus.

Lesions Disruptions in the body's tissues either through injury, as with a cut, or through infection where scar tissues may be formed. Lesions may be internal or external.

Lessor AIDS (LAINS) A term which is falling into disuse which was used to identify patients with oral candidiasis, herpes zoster, idiopathic thrombocytopenia, or generalized lymphadenopathy; but who failed to have the full range of symptoms as called for by the Centers for Disease Control's definition of AIDS.

Leukemia A disease caused by cancer or defects in the bone marrow or lymphatic system, both of which lead to a lack of vital blood cells. In the case of bone marrow, the cells that are reduced in numbers are granulocytes, a type of white blood cell; in the case of the lymphatic system, the ability to produce lymphocytes is impaired or eliminated. As the AIDS virus attacks the lymphatic system and uses it to reproduce itself, the ability of the lymphatic system to make lymphocytes that can still contribute to the body's immune functions is progressively diminished.

Leukocyte White blood corpuscles (including the neutrophils, blastophils and eosindphils) and the granulocytes (lymphocytes and monocytes).

Leukopenia A decrease in the number of white blood cells. The threshold value for leukopenia is usually taken as less than 5000 white blood cells per cubic millimeter of blood.

Leukoplakia A thickening of part of the lining of the mouth or tongue, usually as a result of irritation from a tooth or smoking, but also one of the early indications of cancer of the mouth. A "hairy" leukoplakia lesion in some AIDS patients contains both Papillam avirus and Epstein-Barr viruses.

Listeria monocytogenes (Sp.) A bacteria which can cause meningitis in man and can also infect animals. AIDS patients with listeria respond to treatment.

Lithium carbonate A possible antiviral agent found by David M. Parenti of George Washington Medical Center to be too toxic to be used in more than a limited therapy administered to AIDS cases.

LM427 A new drug that in limited trials has been effective in treating 87 percent of patients with Mycobacterium avium complex.

Lupus erythematosys Inflammation of the connective tissue, particularly the skin, joints, nervous system and muscle membranes of unknown but probably of virus origin.

LTR The long terminal repeat sequence is a component of the AIDS genome.

Lymphadenopathy syndrome (LAS) The failure of the lymphatic system to produce lymphocytes, the white blood cells necessary for the protection of the body against disease. The syndrome may be caused by infection of the lymph with the AIDS virus, HTLV-III, which causes a lymphoma or cancer of the lymph system.

Lymphocyte A white blood cell produced by the lymphatic system that accounts for 30 percent of the white blood cells found in the blood of a healthy individual.

Lymphokine Products of the lymphatic cells which stimulate the production of disease-fighting agents and the activities of other lymphatic cells. Among the lymphokindes are Gamma interferon and interleukin 2.

Lymphoma A malignant cancer of the lymphatic system. These cancers may be caused by infection with the AIDS virus as well as from other causes. Such cancers often spread through the lymphatic system.

Lymphothropic Having to do with the lymphatic system.

Lymph node A lymph node is one of a large number of lymph glands in the body, including the spleen. These glands are connected by lymphatics, small vessels that form a network throughout the body.

Macrophage A "sticky" blood cell which captures and digests foreign substances and presents antigens to the T-cells so that a specific toxic agent to kill or neutralize the foreign material can be produced.

Malaise A feeling of general physical and mental discomfort that is attributable to no particular cause.

Malaria A disease of tropic and semi-tropical regions caused by the infection of the blood-born parasite, Plasmodium, which is transmitted to humans by the bite of the Anopheles mosquito and also by using contaminated needles. Malaria damages the body both from the ravages of high temperature, but, more seriously, by releasing clusters of dead cells into the bloodstream, which may block blood vessels in the kidneys or brain.

Marijuana A plant, Nicotiana glauca, that contains cannabin and has an intoxicating effect when smoked. Marijuana has also been investigated as a possible cofactor in contributing to the onset of AIDS. No conclusive link has been found between the drug and the change of AIDS from a dormant to an advanced stage of the disease. The drug is directly linked with lessening an individual's resistance to participating in unsafe sexual activities which the individual might not otherwise consider.

Meningitis An infection, caused by one or more viruses,

of the membranes, or meninges, surrounding the brain or spinal cord. Herpes simplex or the virus that causes mumps may cause such infections, as may the HTLV-III virus which is responsible for AIDS.

Methadone A synthetic, addictive narcotic used for relieving severe pain and as a substitute for heroin. As a part of drug treatment, a heroin addict may be treated with methadone, which is reduced in dosage until the craving for heroin is reduced.

Microbiology The study of small organisms of a size as are often investigated by using a microscope.

Microcytichypochromic anemia A reduced number of microcytes, the small red blood corpuscles.

Microglial A tissue in the central nervous system that branches from the nerves.

Microglial nodules Knots of tissue found in the spinal cord or brain which in AIDS patients are caused by infection by the AIDS virus and/or <u>Toxoplasma gondii</u>. These nodules and lesions found in the brain are thought to be the cause of the progressive loss of mental powers, or dementia, sometimes observed in people with AIDS.

Microorganisms Any organism that is small enough to require a microscope for identification. There is no lower size limit implied by the use of this term.

Mitogen A substance injected under the skin to determine the functional ability of the body's immune system. Pokeweed and tetanus toxin are commonly used mitogens.

Monoclonal antibodies Antibodies reproduced from clones of a single cell by genes splicing that are targeted for a particular infectious agent.

Monocytes A white blood cell with a single nucleus.

Mononucleosis (Mono) A viral infection giving sore throat-like symptoms with a general feeling of illness and a lack of energy. The onset of mononucleosis mimics some of the general symptoms seen in AIDS. This disease is thought to be caused by the Epstein-Barr virus. The infection yields a large number of mononuclear (single nucleus) white blood cells and an enlargement of the lymph nodes.

Mortality Generally referred to as a death rate. As of April, 1985, there was an accumulated total of 10,000 AIDS cases reported in the U.S. of which 5000 had died for a mortality rate of 50 percent.

Mucosal Having to do with the mucous membranes such as those found in the mouth, respiratory, and digestive tracts. The site of the activity of mucosal lymphocytes and also of some Kaposi's sarcoma infections.

Mucous membranes The linings of the mouth, respiratory, and digestive tracts which secrete fluids to ease the passage of food and waste products and trap infectious particles.

Multinucleated A type of cell which has more than one nucleus. This may be a normal or a cancerous cell.

Mycobacterial drug A drug used in treatment of mycobacterial infections such as that which causes tuberculosis and leprosy.

Mycobacterial tuberculosis A tuberculosis caused by mycobacterial infection, particularly by Mycobacterium tuberculosis.

Mycobacterium avium (Sp.) One of several bacteria which may cause life-threatening infections of the lungs and respiratory systems in AIDS patients, but mild symptoms in healthy individuals. When referred to as Mycobacterium avium complex, it also includes the species Mycobacterium <u>intracellularae</u>. Other members of this group include <u>Mycobacterium</u> <u>fortuitum</u> and <u>Mycobacterium</u> <u>gordonii</u>, both of which may cause disseminated disease in AIDS patients.

Myelitis Inflammation or infection of the myelin sheaths which surround the nerves in the body. In some cases the disease is linked to a viral infection. In advanced cases the disease advances to multiple sclerosis.

Myelopathy Any infection or injury to the spinal cord.

Needlestick injury An injury, typically to health-care personnel, caused by accidentally sticking themselves with a used needle. Disposal of needles into stick-proof containers, rather than attempting to replace them in their original protective sheaths, is recommended for disposable needles.

Neonatal An event occurring at or shortly after birth.

Necropsy An examination made after death.

Neurological complaints Robert L. Levy of the Univ. of California at San Francisco reports that out of 16,576 AIDS cases reported by January of 1986, 7.46 percent reported central nervous system disease with cryptococcosis causing disorders in 4.3 percent of cases; toxoplasmosis, 2.23 percent; progressive multifocal leukoencephalopathy (PML), 0.52 percent; and lymphoma of the central nervous system, 0.48 percent.

Neuropathology The death or disease of part of the nervous system.

Neutropenia A reduced number of neutrophil cells in the blood.

Neurotropism Attracted to or commonly affecting the nerves.

Neutrophil The most common variety of white blood cells, or leukocytes, in the blood.

Nonoxynol-9 A drug commonly used as a spermicide which has also been shown to kill the AIDS virus as well as several other sexually transmitted disease organisms.

Oocysts Immature female gametes of some protozoans, called oocytes, which are passed through the body in small capsules and serve as a means of identifying the protozoan. Cysts may also be formed in the mucus membranes of the body or at sites of infection.

ORF The open reading frame in the AIDS-virus genome.

Opportunistic infections An infectious agent that may occur after the body's immune system has been weakened. Opportunistic infections common in AIDS patients include Pneumocystis carinii pneumonia, Kaposi's sarcoma, shigellosis, histoplasmosis, and other parasitic, viral, and fungal infections, and some types of cancers.

Oralpharyngeal secretions Spit.

Ostracism The isolation of a person from society and his friends, which is a frequent fear of AIDS patients. This fear should be unwarranted as AIDS patients pose no particular hazard to others as long as sexual contact, sharing of blood, or handling body waste products is not involved.

Papillomas Small benign tumors growing on the skin composed of skin tissue and typically covered by it such as corns and warts.

Papillomavirus The virus that causes papillomas. It has also been linked to cancer formation of the genitals.

Papovavirus A virus that causes a severe inflammation, or encephalitis, of the brain. No successful therapy for this viral infection has been developed.

Papule A small, solid tissue-covered protrusion of the skin or mucus membrane.

Parasite An organism that lives on or within a host and derives its nourishment from it.

Parenteral Pertaining to the withdrawal of or introduction of fluids or tissues into the body other than through the digestive system, such as blood being drawn from a vein in the arm or introduced into that vein via a transfusion.

Pasteurization The heating of a material, such as milk or blood products, to the point where organisms within it are killed.

Pathology The examination of dead organisms or of tissue to determine the nature of the disease and/or the cause of death.

PCP (Pneumocystis carinii (Sp.) pneumonia) Infection by this one-celled animal, a protozoan, is the most common opportunistic infection in AIDS patients. The disease is difficult to treat and, once the disease is cured, it may reoccur. This is one of and perhaps the most frequent cause of death of AIDS patients.

Pediatric Having to do with children or their care.

Pediatric AIDS A newly suggested unofficial definition of AIDS in children. Children can be diagnosed as having AIDS with reasonable certainty if they have a persistent gamma globulin anemia, a history of being associated with a risk group, abnormal T-and-B-cell activity and antibodies to the HTLV-III virus. This definition was suggested because children do not often display the usual opportunistic infections of adults needed to define the disease under the criteria used by the Centers for

Disease Control.

Pentamidine isothionate A drug being experimentally used to treat <u>Pneumocystis</u> <u>carinii</u> pneumonia, but which limited use has shown to have a 38 percent toxic response in AIDS patients.

Peripheral Away from the center of an organism or involving the skin or outer covering of the organism.

PGL Persistent generalized lymphadenopathy.

Periorbital Kaposi's sarcoma A type of eye infection caused by Kaposi's sarcoma.

Phagocytes Cells in the reticuloendothelial system and the leukocytes in the bloodstream that consume foreign material and dead cells.

Phenotype 1. A group of organisms sharing the same genetic heritage. 2. Defining a disease by a given set of symptoms.

Platelets A clotting agent in the blood. Platelets are commonly given to those with hemophilia whose blood lacks the clotting agent. Until a Pasteurization process was developed to kill the AID virus in blood products, platelets administered to hemophiliacs was one means of transmitting the AIDS infection.

Pneumocystis carinii (Sp.) pneumonia (PCP) Infection by this one-celled animal, a protozoan, is the most common opportunistic infection in AIDS patients. The disease is difficult to treat, and once the disease is cured, it may reoccur. This is one of, and perhaps the most frequent, cause of death of AIDS patients.

POL The gene containing polymerase that forms a part of the AIDS-virus genome.

Polyacrylamide gel electropheresis (PAGE) A method of determining the protein composition of cells used to identify and determine the structure of the cells.

Pokeweed response A skin test in which an extract of pokeweed, <u>Phytolacca</u> <u>americana</u>, is injected under the skin to determine the ability of the body's immune system to respond. If there is no reddening of the skin near the injection, the immune system is not functioning properly.

Poppers (amphetamines) An often addictive central nervous system stimulant used in pill form as an "upper" to produce extreme energy and unusual excitement. Poppers have been investigated as a cofactor in causing the onset of serious complications resulting from infection with, or exposure to, the AIDS virus. No positive link has been established, but the recreational use of amphetamines among high risk groups is not recommended.

Postmortem After death, often referring to an examination of the body or tissue.

Pre-AIDS A term, that some suggest be discontinued, used to describe certain symptoms of immunosuppression as being a predecessor disease to AIDS. More investigation revealed that there is no one set of clinical symptoms that can, with certainty, predict that a person will develop AIDS.

Premordib pessimism A general non-caring attitude about the prospect of living any longer expressed by someone who knows he is facing a fatal illness.

Psychological Having to do with a person's mental responses to himself, his environment, and to ideas.

Psychosocial A combination of psychological and sociological approaches to treat those who may have potentially fatal illnesses, like AIDS. This approach considers not only the person's mental well being but also his activities in society and the response of society to him.

PWA People with AIDS, particularly the National Association of People With AIDS based in Washington, D.C.

Pyrimethamine A drug used by F. Raffi of the Claude Bernard Hospital in Paris to cure <u>Toxoplasma gondii</u> infections. In a trial of 35 patients at the hospital, the drug improved the condition of 88.5 percent of the trial cases.

Quaaludes An amphetamine in pill form that is common as an illegal drug.

Quarantine The enforced confinement of those with a communicable disease.

Radioimmunoassay A method of protein analysis and identification at the cell level which identifies the protein by binding hormones with short-lived radioactive tracers to a specific antibody. The antibody attaches itself to the particular protein being sought, enabling the proteins to be counted by radiation detector.

Renal Having to do with the kidneys.

Reticuloendothelial system A system of interstitial cells that includes all the phagocytic cells which trap and consume foreign agents, except the leukocytes circulating in the bloodstream. This system forms a network throughout the body and is another of the body's defense systems against invading organisms in the connective tissues of the body.

Retinal hemorrhage Bleeding inside the eye which may be caused by an injury or in AIDS patients by Kaposi's sarcoma or virus infections.

Retinitis Inflammation of the retina of the eye which may be caused in AIDS patients by Kaposi's sarcoma.

Retrovirus This is the family of viruses that includes HTLV-III, the virus that causes AIDS, as well as other viruses that attack mice, chickens, cats, sheep, cattle and other mammals. Viruses of the retrovirus family frequently have a long incubation period after the initial infection before the disease becomes apparent. Some retroviruses produce spreading cancerous or malignant diseases, some both malignant and nonmalignant diseases, and some only nonmalignant diseases.

Reverse transcriptase A DNA synthesizing enzyme found in retroviruses. The amount of reverse transcriptase in a sample indicates the number of infecting viruses and how rapidly they are reproducing.

Rheumatoid arthritis This is thought to be an autoimmune disease where the body's own immune system is attacking and inflaming a thin membrane surrounding the joints. Persons with arthritis are known to have "sticky antibodies" which may sometimes give false positive tests for AIDS with some techniques.

Ribivirin An antiviral drug which in limited tests appears to be effective against the AIDS virus. This is one of the more expensive of the new drugs used against AIDS with a three-day supply of the drug reported to cost $687.

Rifapertine A drug in first test in mice that may be effective against Mycobacterium avium pneumonia.

Rimming The tongue of one sex partner contacting and penetrating the anus of another.

Risk group A segment of the population that is at increased risk for contracting a particular disease. In the case of AIDS high risk groups include gays, bisexuals, intravenous drug abusers, sexual partners of those who later developed AIDS, prostitutes, those with a large number of sex partners, hemophiliacs, and those who have received frequent blood transfusions within the last three to five years.

Salmonella (salmonellosis) A bacterial infection of the digestive system that causes diarrhea. Salmonella is most frequently contracted through meat that has been improperly cooked or thawed. It is possible for the body to host the bacteria even after the symptoms have passed. Salmonellosis is another of the opportunistic diseases which may affect AIDS patients. One species, Salmonella typhoneurium, causes symptoms similar to typhoid fever.

Sarcoma A cancer of the mesodermal tissues of the body which may include connective tissue, bone, cartilage, or muscle. A type of sarcoma, Kaposi's sarcoma, is common among AIDS patients.

Seminal fluid The fluid discharged from the penis which contains the male sperm as well as lubricating and nourishing agents. This fluid is the most common media by which the AIDS virus is spread.

Sepsis The spread of a bacterial infection from its entry point and the accumulation of bacterial and waste products around the site of the infection into the bloodstream and/or lymphatic system.

Septic episodes Infectious episodes.

Sera 1. Fluids, usually blood, drawn for examination. 2. Any of a number of preparations used to culture cell growth or extracts from cell cultures.

Suramin An antiviral drug which in culture and patient testing has shown itself capable of killing the AIDS virus, but which also has serious side effects. The drug functions by inhibiting the production of reverse transcriptase, a substance needed for the virus to reproduce.

Serology   The investigation and examination of sera and also the science of investigating sera.

Seroepidemiological   The investigation of an epidemic by the extraction and examination of sera (blood or other materials) from those exposed to the infectious agent.

Seroincidence The frequency of seroconversion.

Seronegative   As used to indicate the results of ELISA testing for the AIDS virus, a seronegative response indicates that the test detected no antibodies to the AIDS virus in that portion of the sample that was tested. This is an ambiguous results and may indicate that the HTLV-III virus is latent and the body is not producing antibodies to it, that the virus is a new infection and the body has not had sufficient time to produce antibodies, or that the patient's immune system has failed due to AIDS or other diseases and can produce no antibodies to the infectious agent.   A seronegative response does not positively prove that the person being tested is "safe" and cannot transmit AIDS to another, but it does indicate that a seronegative person has a higher probability of not having the AIDS virus than one whose test results are seropositive.

Seropositive   A seropositive response to the ELISA test for AIDS indicates that the person being tested is producing antibodies to the HTLV-III virus, which is the infectious agent which causes AIDS.   Because the body of the tested person is producing such antibodies, it is presumed that the person is infected with the virus. The ELISA test, as presently administered, yields a small number of false-positive results, and all seropositives should be reassayed by another type of test to insure that the seropositive result is correct. Seropositivity does not mean that the person being tested will develop AIDS, but it is generally assumed that such a person is capable of transmitting the virus to others by having sexual relations with transfer of body fluids, using contaminated needles, and through blood products.

Shigella flexneri (Sp.) A species of bacteria that causes severe dysentery which may last for a year or more with up to 20 bowel movements per day. When this dysentery is proved to be caused by the bacteria, the disease infection is called shigellosis. A related bacteria, Shigella sonnei, causes similar symptoms. Antibiotic treatment has proved to be effective if the disease is not also complicated by a simultaneous infection of cytomegalovirus which does not respond to antibiotics.

Shooting gallery A place where injectable drugs are illegally sold.

SIDA The abbreviation for AIDS expressed in French, Spanish, and other Romance Languages.

Social alienation The effective removal of a person from his former group of friends and associates because of a disease, condition or change in social status which leads to the person's feeling that he is unwanted by society.

Sodium phosphonoformate A drug which inhibits reverse transcriptase activity of the AIDS virus.

SOR The short open reading frame of the AIDS virus genome.

Southern blot See Western blot.

Spiramycin A drug used with limited success to control cryptosporidiosis.

Spleen The largest lymphatic organ in the body. It is located in the upper left abdomen behind the ribs.

Squamous carcinoma of the tongue A cancer of the tongue which may be linked to the sexual transmission of papillomavirus.

STLV-III   A T-4 cell lymphotrophic virus found in monkeys. The simian AIDS virus.

Streptococcus pneumonia   A type of pneumonia caused by infection by the streptococcus bacteria. Most often streptococcus infections affect the skin, throat, or kidneys; but in AIDS patients, pneumonia may also result from streptococcus infection.

Streptomycin   An antibiotic drug commonly used for treatment of the bacterial infection which causes tuberculosis, but ineffective against bacterial infections caused by <u>Mycobacterium</u> <u>avium</u> complex in AIDS patients.

Subcortial dementia   A dementia, or loss of reasoning abilities, caused by a pathologic illness or infection of the lower brain.

Suramin   A drug which first had promising results in inhibiting the growth of the AIDS virus, but was reported by Lawrence D. Kaplan of San Francisco General to be "ineffective therapy for AIDS patients and to have significant toxicity."

TAT   The transactivating transcription gene found in the genome of the AIDS virus. The TAT gene was found by Amanda Fisher of the National Cancer Institute to be linked to the long terminal repeat sequence of the AIDS virus and to be necessary for virus reproduction.

Thrombocytopenia   A deficiency in the numbers of platelets in the blood.

T-4 lymphocytes   The T-4 lymphocytes are the chief cells attacked by the AIDS virus. Once they become cancerous, their reproductive machinery is taken over by the HTLV-III virus, and the cells lose their capacity to produce antibodies to combat infectious agents. In advanced stages of AIDS few antibodies to the virus will be found in blood samples because of the increasing inability of the lymphocytes to function.

Thalassemia A hereditary blood disease in which the body does not produce sufficient hemoglobin. Frequent trans-fusions are necessary to restore the blood's ability to carry oxygen to the body's cells.

Thiobendazole A drug used in therapy against the round-worm <u>Strongyliodes stercoralis</u>.

Tetanus (lockjaw) This bacterial infection is usually caused by a puncture wound penetrating the skin, allowing soil-living bacteria to enter the body. Unless the body is immunized to the tetanus toxin, tetanus attacks the nerve cells in the body, leading to muscle spasms and perhaps suffocation because of muscle spasms of the throat or chest. Tetanus toxin is also used as one of the standard skin tests to determine the effectiveness of the body's immune system.

Trimethoprim – sulfamethoxazole A drug suggested for use against PCP, but its high toxicity was found by Lawrence D. Kaplan to preclude its use as a PCP prophylaxis in AIDS.

Thrombocytopenia A deficiency in the number of blood platelets.

Tropism The tendency of a virus or other organism to prefer a particular host.

Thrush Sore patches in the mouth caused by the fungi <u>Candida albicans</u>. Thrush is one of the most frequent early symptoms of an immune disorder. The fungi commonly lives in the mouth, but only causes problems when the body's resistance is reduced either by antibiotics which have reduced the number of competitive organisms in the mouth or by an immune deficiency.

Thymus A gland in the upper chest at the base of the

neck which is part of the lymphatic system and the produ-
cer of T-cells.

Titers A measure of the concentration of a material
expressed in amount, or percent, per unit of fluid.
Sometimes less precisely used to express a general high
or low amount of material in solution.

Toxic dose A dosage of medication or poison sufficient
to kill the person or organism to which it is administered.

Toxicity The ability of a substance to poison an organism.

Toxoplasma gondii (Sp.) A protozoan parasite that is
the cause of toxoplasmosis in man and is thought to be a
major cause of brain damage in AIDS patients.

Toxoplasmosis A disease caused by a toxoplasma infection
which may give rise to pneumonia, hepatitis, or encephalitis, but particularly to lesions and brain damage in
AIDS patients. This is a common infection, but as a
disease is uncommon except in patients whose immune system is not functional.

Trimethoprim sulfamethoxazole (bactrim) A combination of
two drugs sold under the brand name Bactrim that is used
in treatment of Pneumocystis carinii pneumonia. For those
who can tolerate the drug, a favorable response has been
reported in some cases in as few as 10 days. Toxic side
effects were observed for some patients.

Trypanosomiasis Sleeping sickness, which in Africa is
caused by Trypanosoma gambiense and in North America by
Trypanosoma cruzi.

Tuberculosis A disease of the lungs caused by bacterial
infection.

Vaginal-cervical secretions Secretions of the woman's genitals which have been found to contain the AIDS virus.

VD Any sexually transmitted disease.

Vinblastine A drug extracted from the periwinkle, <u>Vinca rosea</u>, used to treat malignant tumors. In human trials, patients have noted lessened pain and gained weight. This drug has also been used to treat Hodgkin's disease and in chemotherapeutic treatment of Kaposi's sarcoma and lymphatic cancers.

Viral Having to do with viruses, as in a viral infection.

Viremia Infection by a virus.

Virus Any of a very large number of disease-causing submicroscopic organisms that are capable of growth and multiplication only in living cells. They are composed of complex proteins having a variety of external, often crystal-like, forms. Viruses are much smaller than cells.

Visna (visnavirus) A type of lentiretrovirus that infects animals which has similar characteristics to the AIDS virus. This virus also infects the central nervous system and has a long incubation period.

Vitro To be grown or cultured in glass containers, as in a laboratory test of a drug.

Vivo To be tested with animal, usually human, subjects.

Walter Reed classification A system of AIDS classification developed by the U.S. Army which ranges from WR0, high risk exposure, to WR6, invasive opportunistic infections.

Watersports Sexual play involving urine.

Western blot A test made with a gel to determine the

reactivity of certain protein antibodies to electrical current. Antibodies produced in response to the AIDS virus can be detected using this technique. Sometimes called Southern Blot after the name of the originator of the test, a Dr. Southern.

Zaire A country in Central Africa, formerly the Belgian Congo.

Zairian A native of Zaire.

INDEX

REPORTED INFECTIONS

Viral Infections
   Adenovirus
   Cytomegalovirus
   Epstein-Barr virus
   Herpes simplex virus
   Papovavirus
   Varicella (Herpes)-zoster

Fungal Infections
   Aspergillis (Sp.)
   Candida albicans
   Candida tropicalis
   Cryptococcus neoformans
   Histoplasma capsulatum

Bacterial Infections

Clostridium perfringens
Haemophilus influenzae
Isospora belli
Legionella (Sp.)
Listeria monocytogenes
Pseudomonas aeruginosa
Mycobacterium avium
Mycobacterium fortuitum
Mycobacterium gordonae
Mycobacterium intracellulare
Mycobacterium tuberculosis

Mycobacterium xenopi
Nocardia asteroides
Salmonella enteriditis
Salmonella typhimurium
Salmonella (Sp.)
Shigalla (Sp.)
Staphylococcus aureus
Staphylococcus epidermidis
Staphylococcus pneumoniae

Parasitic Infections

Cryptosporidium (Sp.)
Entamoeba histolytica
Giardia lamblia

Pneumocystis carinii
Strongyloides stercoralis
Toxoplasma gondii

AIDS NEWSLETTERS

WEEKLY

CDC AIDS WEEKLY A private, non-government weekly publication edited by Charles Henderson. $520 a year. 1409 Fairview Road, Atlanta Georgia 30306.

MONTHLY

AIDS ALERT A private monthly newsletter published by American Health Consultants. $79 per year. AIDS ALERT, Dept. 4908, 67 Peachtree Park Drive, N.E., Atlanta, Georgia 30309.

THE NAN NEWSLETTER Published by the National AIDS Network, this bi-monthly publication is distributed to members as a part of membership services. Memberships are available to concerned individuals, health care providers, businesses, corporations, and organizations. For membership applications and current fees inquire to: National AIDS Network, 729 8th Street, S.E., Washington D.C. 20003.

WORKS BY THE AUTHOR

Geology of the Tennille Lime Sinks, Washington County, Georgia: 1983, 32 p., ills., glossary. An introduction to the origin of caves and the Eocene fossils of Georgia..$3.50

Kaolin Deposits of Central Georgia: An Introduction to Their Origin and Use: 1983, 96 p., ills., glossary, index. The first comprehensive work on Central Georgia's kaolin industry published in more than 50 years.....$6.50

Guide to Homes and Plantations of the Thomasville (Georgia) Region: 1984, 60 p., ills., index. An architectural guide that also examines the changing life of southwest, rural Georgia during the last 150 years..$5.50

Farnagle's Fables for Children and Adults: 1984, 61 p., ills., story guides. Four original stories, "Alphred, the Purple-horned Snail," "The Frog Who Would Stop Winter," "War of the Spotted Ants," and "The Not So Goody Gum Drop Shop" with story guides examine moral and social issues in a form that is palatable to children......$4.25

"The Not So Goody Gum Drop Shop - A Play in One Act:" 1984, 23 p. A play warning of the dangers of drug abuse designed for presentation by a mixed-age cast......$3.50

Guide to the Geology of Bartow County, Georgia: 1985, 44p. ills., index. A treatment of the geologic evolution of a Northwest Georgia county important for its production of barite, iron, manganese, and aluminum, including a general history of mineral development...........$5.00

Plain Words About AIDS: 1985, (First Edition) 132 p., ills., glossary, index. A presentation of the syndrome based on papers from the 1985 International Conference on

AIDS, releases from the Centers for Disease Control through September 13, 1985, and articles from the national wire services through October 10, 1985....$10.00

Plain Words About AIDS: 1985, (Second Edition) 200 p., ills., glossary, index. A presention of the syndrome from the 1986 Second International Conference on AIDS in Paris, releases from the Centers for Disease Control through July 4, 1986, and articles from the national wire services through October 20, 1986.................$17.50

Muzzle Loading Through Georgia, 1986, (In Progress) Why, how, and where to hunt and shoot with muzzle-loading arms in Georgia including the humorous adventures of the Skunk Hollow Muzzle-Loading Club.

Available From

WHITEHALL PRESS-BUDGET PUBLICATIONS
Whitehall
Rte. 1   Box 603
Sandersville, Georgia 31082

362.1
SMI

3/27/95

Smith, Wm. Hovey, ed.
Aids; plain words about.

DATE	BORROWER'S NAME	ROOM NUMBER

362.1
SMI

PB

Smith, Wm. Hovey, ed.
Aids; plain words about.

This book may be kept
FOURTEEN DAYS

**A fine will be charged for each
day the book is kept overtime.**

11/11/94			

HIGHSMITH 45—226